ADVANCE PRAISE

"In these days of political correctness and, for some, keeping your opinions to yourself lest you get a tirade of angry comments, it is refreshing to hear the voice of Theresa Wee. She fearlessly voices her expertise, her stories, and her opinions on things that matter to her. She is the voice of a working mother raising four children. She is the voice of one who has lost her spouse. She is the voice of one who is reconnecting to God. She is the voice in the wilderness, suggesting that we can overcome, we can change the direction of our lives by making the right choices."

—PASTOR JERRY HIGASHI, MOMILANI
CHRISTIAN CHURCH, PEARL CITY, HAWAII

"Dr. Wee has been a great inspiration to me during this 'unprecedented' year, 2020. She freely shares her heart, personal life experiences, faith in God, and her knowledgeable medical expertise with anyone. She has been a source of great hope for many, and I am extremely grateful for her friendship. I always look forward to seeing her every Sunday, and I know you will also feel the same when you read this book."

—CYNTHIA MURATA, RETIREE

"When COVID-19 hit us last year, we were all suddenly stuck at home. As one of the weekly attendees to her "Walk with a Doc – Oahu" event, I greatly missed her energy, enthusiasm, and infectious smile. Lucky for all of us, she decided to start writing a daily blog at the beginning of lockdown. For me, these blogs have not only been entertaining, but more importantly, they have been uplifting and inspiring. With her wisdom and knowledge, she educates and challenges us to be the best we can be. She probably has no idea how many people she has touched, but I know her love and dedication have improved countless lives. I am grateful to have such a caring friend. She is my hero!"

—RENATA RIVERA, RETIREE

"Who can forget the year 2020 and how this coronavirus affected each one of us? We all went through turmoil and uncertainty during this worldwide COVID-19 pandemic. However, through the stories and experiences that Dr. Wee shared, she not only offers valuable tips for dealing with difficult situations but also reveals how her faith in God continues to sustain her through even the darkest of times. In times like these, it is comforting to know that we can find hope and peace through God, our Heavenly Father. It's an easy read and you won't be able to put this book down!"

—JENNIE LUE, RETIRED OCCUPATIONAL THERAPIST

"I'm so happy that Dr. Wee decided to put her blogs into book form so more people would have an opportunity to spend time with her. She has a natural writing style that makes you feel as though you're visiting with her over a cup of morning coffee. As you read this book, you can see her working through her struggles during the pandemic. What I love most is that she closes each day's blog with a scripture reading that expresses her faith, and this has greatly inspired me to keep moving forward."
—MARY BRETSCHNEIDER, COMMUNITY VOLUNTEER

MY COVID-19 DIARY

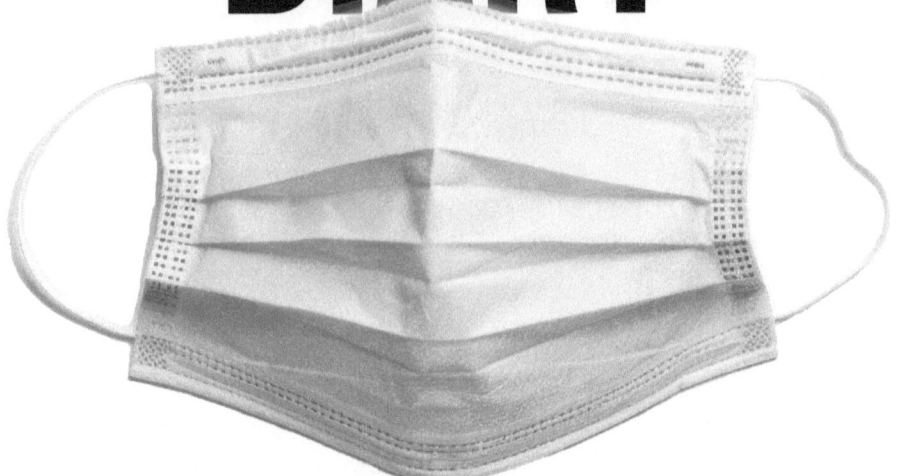

PRACTICAL TIPS AND SCRIPTURES FOR IMPROBABLE TIMES FROM
AN AMERICAN DOCTOR

THERESA Y. WEE, M.D.

Ordering Information:

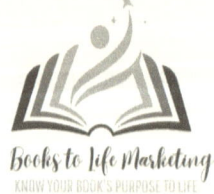

Books to Life Marketing
KNOW YOUR BOOK'S PURPOSE TO LIFE

Books to Life Marketing Ltd
128 City Road, London, EC1V 2NX, UK

Printed in the United States of America

CONTENTS

This book is dedicated to the frontline health care workers worldwide who lost their lives to the COVID-19 virus. They worked tirelessly to help their patients and then gave the ultimate sacrifice, their lives in the line of duty....

We will never forget these heroic healthcare workers and their families, who continue to feel the ripple effects of their lost loved ones.

"Even though I walk through the darkest valley, I will fear no evil, for you are with me, your rod and your staff they comfort me."

—PSALM 23:4 NIV

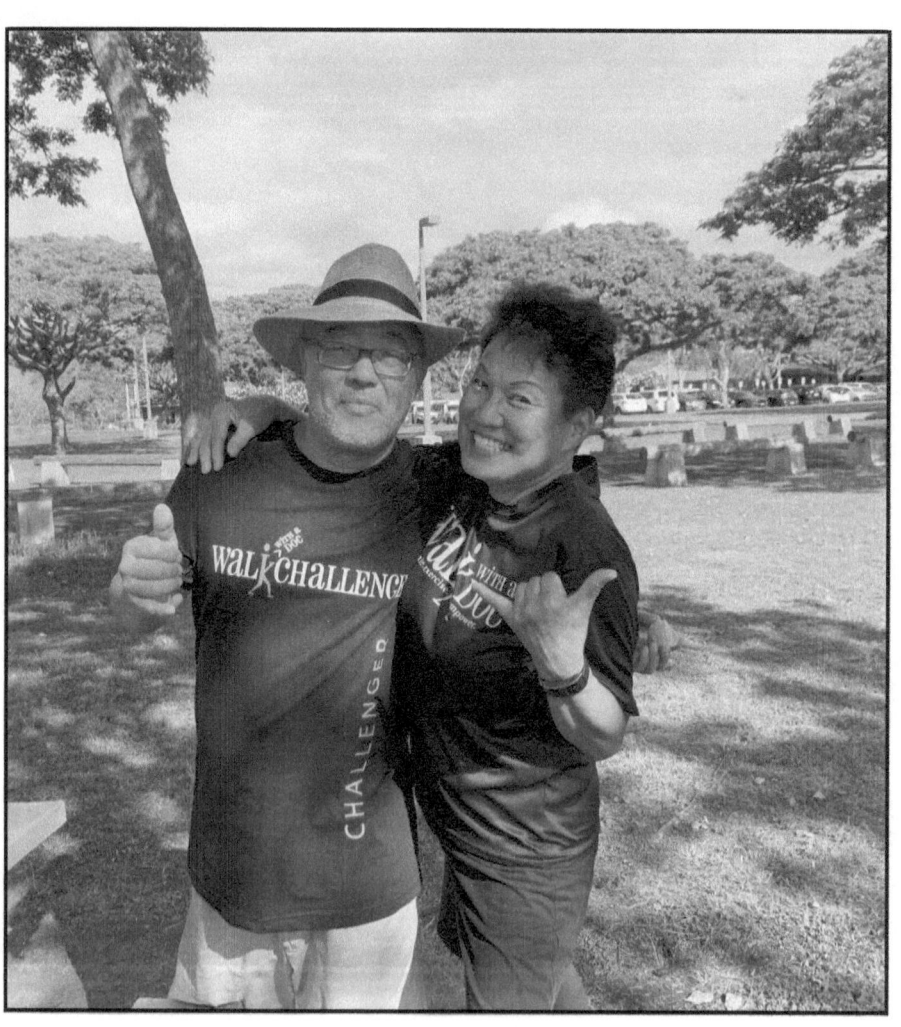

FOREWORD

"Don't slow me down!"

—DR. THERESA WEE

As her husband, I selected these words because they succinctly captured Dr. Theresa Wee's attitude. The COVID-19 pandemic suddenly slammed the brakes on the momentum of life for most people worldwide. The sudden availability of time and pent-up energy caused by stay-at-home orders and the cancellation of many social events due to new social distancing rules was redirected into Theresa's blogs. I, along with many of our friends and family, have enjoyed receiving a peek into her heart and mind. Based on the many positive reactions to these daily blogs, she decided to turn them into a book and make them available to a broader audience, so that you, too, can enjoy these snippets of our 2020 reality through Theresa's eyes.

As a reader, I can say that her personal and transparent writing style offers valuable and practical insights that help to develop a better attitude and have a positive impact on our community. Suppose you're facing challenges in your life. In that case, you'll find inspiration in this collection of daily journal entries, as Theresa has an unparalleled talent for encouraging others with her personal experiences in areas such as medical advice, relationships, raising a family, health tips, overcoming grief, and nurturing faith. Her journal reveals a very personal response during a worldwide pandemic. This book is easy to read and is refreshingly honest.

The pages of this book contain the essence of Theresa. She is highly competitive and has no pushover. She refuses to fall into the victim mentality. She is passionate about addressing the epidemic of childhood obesity and advocates that prevention and family involvement are key to the solution. Theresa is on a mission to make the world a better place. A revolution starts with one person, then a second, and grows to a third. I'm *in* as a second. Will you join us and be the third?

—MARTIN ARINAGA,
CERTIFIED FINANCIAL PLANNER™ PROFESSIONAL,
CO-FOUNDER, CHINEN & ARINAGA FINANCIAL GROUP, INC.
PROUD HUSBAND OF DR. THERESA WEE

AUTHOR'S NOTE

January 2020 beckoned the start of a new decade, and what an exciting time it was for me. I had just completed my first book in 2019, *The Happy, Healthy Revolution: A Parent's Guide to Achieve Wellness as a Family Unit,* and it was now released as an eBook. I looked forward to recording it as an audiobook during the summer of 2020.

As a pediatrician with over forty years of experience and now a bestselling author, I have many exciting and ambitious plans to share my expertise and knowledge through workshops, as well as my newly published book. However, this was not to be, as the new COVID-19 virus began to emerge.

By March 2020, the COVID-19 virus outbreak had become a worldwide pandemic, and now this far-off virus was affecting each one of us here at home. I saw panic, fear, and confusion everywhere, and there was talk of local hospitals not being able to handle all the critically ill patients. There was suddenly much discussion about "flattening the curve," which meant slowing down the rapid spread of this virus so our front-line workers and hospitals could accommodate and care for every critically ill person affected.

As a medical consultant for several area preschools, I began to get frantic calls and requests to answer questions from teachers, administrators, parents, and even the local media. Even in my private practice, I could sense the same type of panic and fear building up daily.

We had never faced a problem like this before, and there were no established protocols. From our top officials in Washington, D.C., to our local politicians, health officials, and infectious disease specialists, the advice was confusing and constantly changing. Cleaning supplies, along with other essentials, were suddenly becoming scarce due to the widespread panic.

Leading up to the lockdown, I was experiencing a range of emotions. First, there was fear, then anger, and finally confusion and frustration over this entire situation, as well as the lack of consistent medical advice that made sense.

Schools began closing completely and transitioning to virtual learning. Finally, on March 23, 2020, it became official that Oahu was going into "lockdown" to contain the rapidly rising COVID-19 cases.

Feelings of worry and anger were taking root in all of us and appeared to be here to stay. I'm not the one to sit back and watch chaos unfold. This was an unprecedented time for all of us, and we needed to hold on tight and get through this together. On the first day of this lockdown, I decided to share my thoughts and feelings in a daily blog, allowing me to continue communicating with family and friends.

Although I had never written daily blogs on social media before, I decided to do so for at least one month. I was eager to share my daily journal of events and thoughts for the day, and by doing so, I hoped to add a little bit of hope and optimism to someone's day.

After writing for a month, I received numerous positive feedback and comments. My faithful blog readers urged me to keep writing. People told me they felt encouraged, and some even looked forward to the daily blogs, like their daily newspaper. I decided to continue writing.

This book is a compendium of my original blogs from March 23, 2020, to December 31, 2020, developed and edited to convey the lessons and insights the pandemic bestowed upon me. I hope that you will gain insight into – not only the turmoil of this time – but also the hope, encouragement, and lessons learned from this journey. I have included practical tips for persevering through this challenging time, along with biblical scriptures that have helped me deepen my faith. I hope this book will help you navigate any bumps in the road you encounter along your own life's journey.

My Heavenly Father continues to sustain and bless me during these uncertain times. I will hold on to my faith as I move forward into an uncertain 2021. 2020 has been a year of unceasing praying for God's wisdom and blessings amidst fear and uncertainty. As one of His children, I will continue to pray and trust that He hears me and already knows what I need even before I ask.

"Be strong and courageous. Do not be afraid or terrified because of them, for the Lord your God goes with you; he will never leave you nor forsake you."

—DEUTERONOMY 31:6 NIV

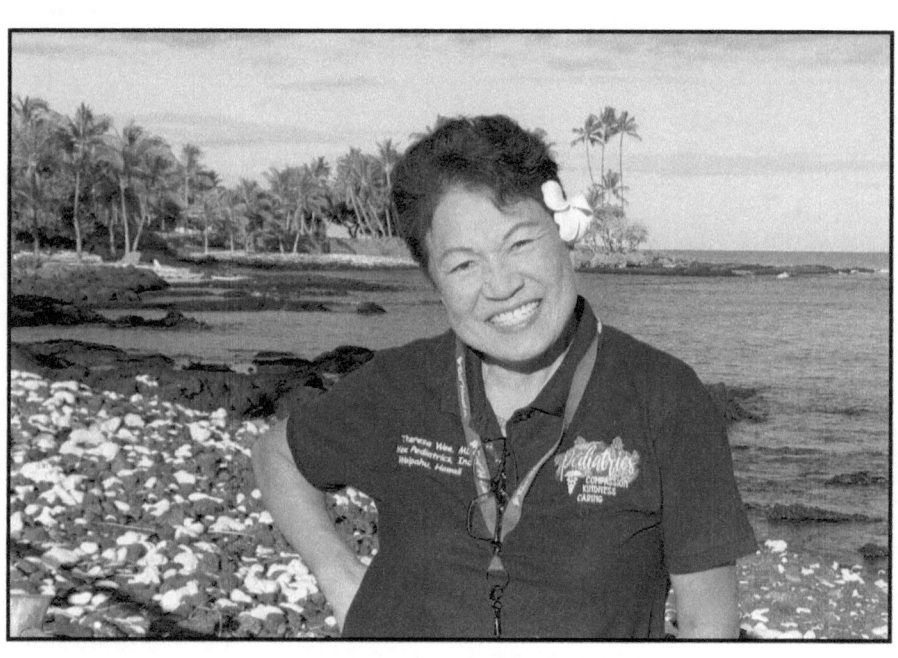

1

MARCH

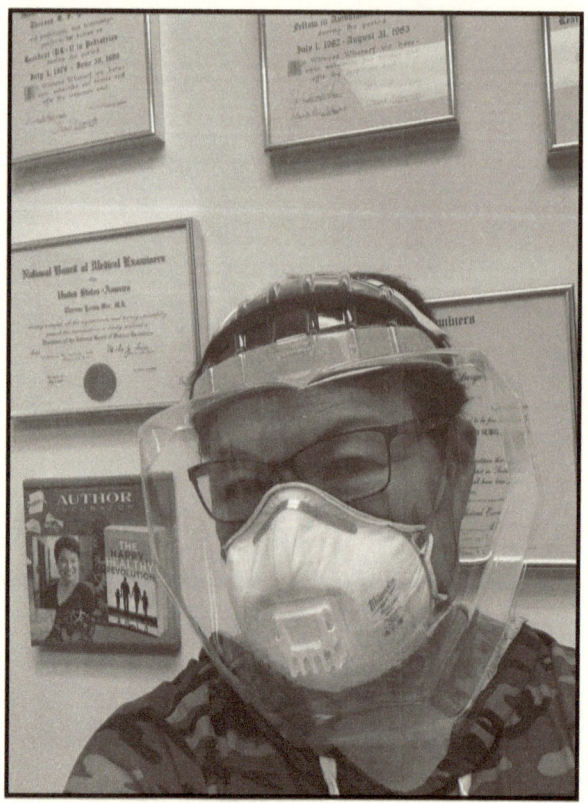

Today is the first day of lockdown for the city and county of Honolulu, Hawaii. As a pediatrician, I continue to see patients in my office. My staff and doctors, as well as I, all began wearing personal protective equipment (PPEs) as recommended by the Centers for Disease Control (CDC). This has been an extremely stressful time for me, not only as a physician but also as a business owner.

I want to continue serving my patients and their families to the best of my ability, while also ensuring the safety and well-being of everyone in my office. I must keep the doors open for as long as possible, but the bills keep coming, and the revenues are declining.

As I write my first blog, I want to remind everyone that we must do our part in minimizing the spread of this deadly virus. We need to wash our hands and keep social distancing first and foremost. We have already seen what has happened in other countries when individuals do not heed this warning. An excellent example of this was in Brazil, where officials never instituted a lockdown. People ignored warnings, and as a result, it became the second most coronavirus-ravaged country in the world. Please think of others who are vulnerable to this deadly virus, such as the elderly, the immunocompromised, and those with underlying medical conditions. You may be able to weather this COVID-19 virus, but someone else may not, and it could be a loved one.

I hope that we all "hunker down," as hard as this may be, this too shall pass. If we see little spread and no deaths in Hawaii, then we will have accomplished our goal of keeping the number of COVID-19 infections to a minimum.

I plan to spend quality time with my dear husband, Martin Arinaga. We will finally be able to tackle home projects that were on hold for months, and even years. I'm also looking forward to taking long, leisurely walks with him and pausing to enjoy the beauty of Hawaii.

We plan on FaceTiming our children, grandchildren, and friends frequently. Additionally, I hope to stay in touch with you, my dear blog readers, through these daily blogs and share my journey as we navigate the challenges of this pandemic together.

> *"But those who hope in the Lord will renew their strength. They will soar on wings like eagles; they will run and not grow weary; they will walk and not be faint."*

> —ISAIAH 40:31 NIV

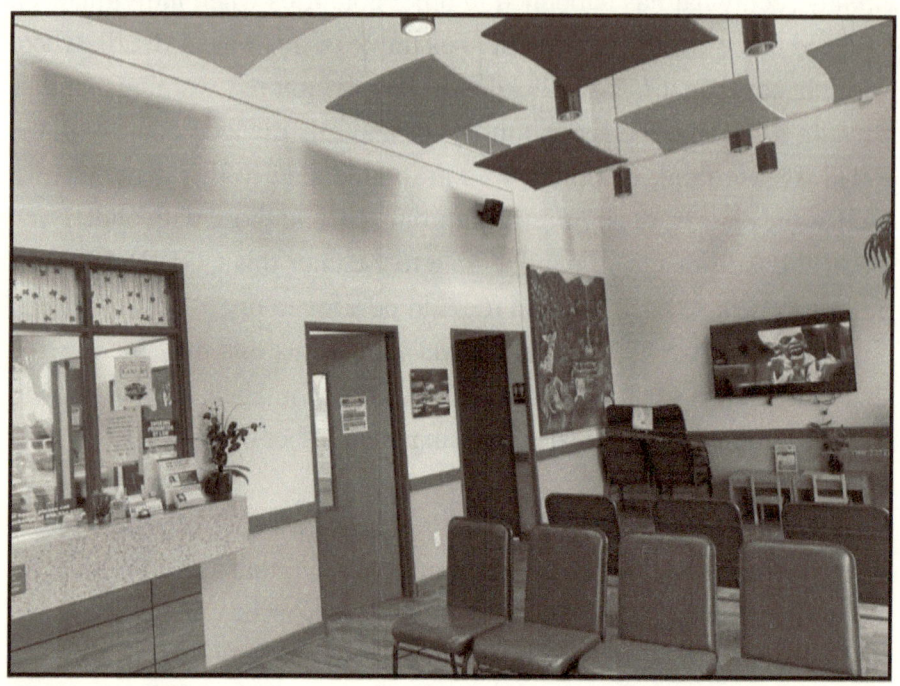

Governor Ige announced that starting tomorrow, the state of Hawaii would be under a statewide "stay-at-home/ work-from-home" order. Life, as we know, is changing, whether we like it or not. But, dear readers, please remember that you are not alone. We are all in this together, and we will get through it.

I continue to see patients in my office, but with slightly shortened hours. We continue to screen each sick call, and the doctor makes a final determination of whether it is vital to see this person in the office. We are working to minimize the risk of infection for our other patients and staff as much as possible. Our well-child visits and vaccine administration continue as usual, so that no one falls behind.

I want to put a reminder out there for folks using "911." Remember, this hotline is for life-threatening emergency calls only. Additionally, I have been receiving an increased number of night calls requesting COVID-19 testing.

If an after-hours call is not an emergency and you can wait until morning, please allow your healthcare provider to get their sleep and call the office in the morning.

Finally, I wanted to remind everyone that boosting your immune system is probably the most crucial way to prevent illness.

Here are some great ways for people of all ages to boost their immune system:

- Keep to a regular schedule.
- Continue with daily activities, such as walking or other physical activities.
- Eat three healthy meals and limit snacks to a minimum.
- Drink lots of water throughout the day.
- Get adequate sleep.
- Stay connected with others frequently via FaceTime or give friends and relatives a call.
- Pause and consider your breathing. Be mindful of the present moment.

So, dear readers, consider this final statement about living in the moment. This is the only time we must modify our actions and decisions. Let's take each day and its burdens as they come because that's all we can ever do. Worry turns to stress, and stress then weakens our immune system.

"Therefore, do not worry about tomorrow, for tomorrow will worry about itself. Each day has enough trouble of its own."

—MATTHEW 6:34 NIV

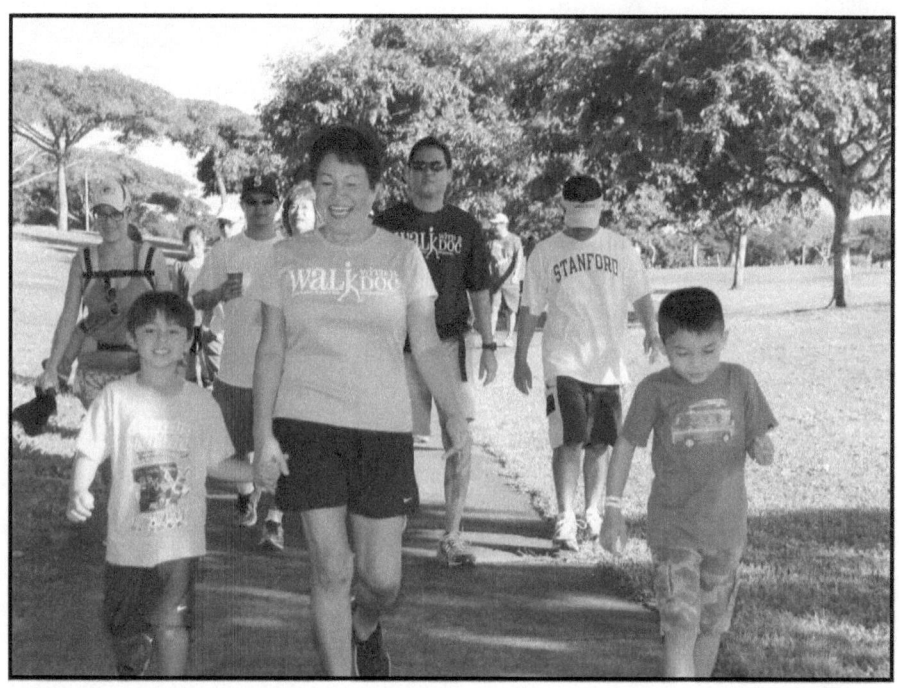

just got through listening to a live televised news conference by our Governor.... Noticeably absent, once again,

It was Lieutenant Governor Josh Green, who was put in charge of Hawaii's COVID-19 pandemic response. Dr. Green is a dear friend and colleague, as well as an ER physician. He needs to be in the forefront once again. Let's not play political games and risk people's lives. I believe he is the most knowledgeable person to coordinate our response, and we need the most qualified individual in our state to lead us.

In other news, I had to close my office completely today. It was a difficult decision to make; however, due to the lack of appointments and financial considerations, I was forced to do so. I hope this will not be a regular occurrence, but right now, it is about balancing the needs of my patients with keeping my business afloat during this pandemic, for however long it lasts.

I spent the morning doing home chores, followed by thirty minutes of intense exercise via live video from my CrossFit Waipio Studio. I was extremely proud of myself for making the most of my time today.

What I realized early in this pandemic is that we now suddenly have an abundance of free time available to all of us. So, dear readers, instead of going through each day aimlessly or spending hours scrolling through our social media feeds, let's try to make the most of each precious day. This pandemic has afforded us precious time. When you stop and think about it, time is our most precious asset. For many people, the common belief is that money is our greatest asset, but no matter how much money you have, if you have no time to enjoy it, then it means nothing.

Let me share with you some tips I've come up with to make the most of our day. First, have a general plan or goals in mind at the start of the day and begin your day with intention. By this, I mean staying connected to what truly matters to you and choosing actions that align with your genuine purpose. Be aware of your time wasters, such as Facebook, playing video games, watching movies, online shopping, and other activities that consume your time. Instead, free up your time and go through your day being proactive instead of reactive. Finally, remember that our time here on Earth is limited, so make the most of the time God has given us.

> *"Why, you do not even know what will happen tomorrow. What is your life? You are a mist that appears for a little while and then vanishes."*
>
> —JAMES 4:14 NIV

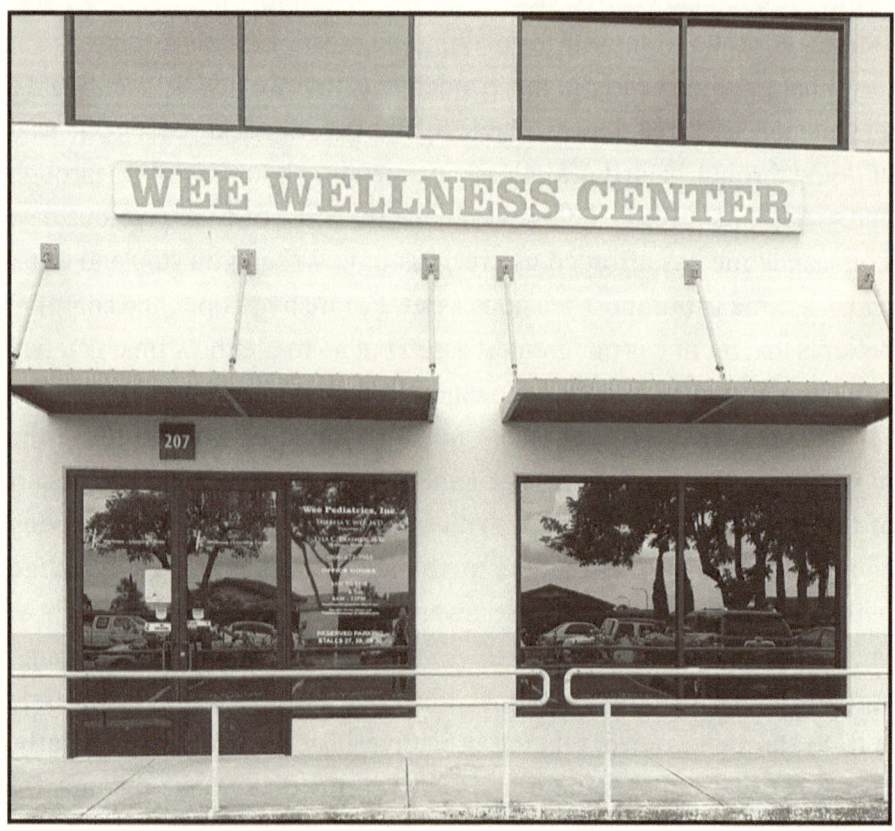

T oday, I worked in the office to see my patients. Many of the visits continue to be mainly well-child visits with vaccine updates. We have had a handful of selected sick visits in the office, as most are being handled over the phone. Patients and parents have been very understanding and flexible as we navigate this unusual pandemic. I huddle with my team nearly every day as we try to adjust to the constantly changing recommendations. I wear all my protective gear with every patient visit, which includes an N95 face mask, a large face shield, a coat, and glasses. It is extremely hot, difficult to breathe, and my glasses and face shield are constantly fogging up. At the end of my shift, I was dripping sweat, but I made it through seeing everyone. There were no cancellations today, and I believe many folks welcomed this little respite to come out of home quarantine and see their primary care physician.

It was very heartwarming to hear comments of appreciation for keeping our office open. I have the best staff and feel very blessed to have such a great team. If you have a family member or friend in the healthcare field, please take a moment to express your gratitude for their service during these challenging times. As healthcare workers, we expose ourselves to the COVID-19 virus daily while serving our community. This is what we have been trained to do all our lives.

April 30, 2020, seems like a long time away, but I'll do my best to social distance, wash my hands, and wear all the protective equipment as directed. This pandemic has affected all of us in a very extreme way, but we'll get through this together.

Take a moment to cherish this precious time spent connecting with family members. Sit down and enjoy family meals, play a board game, or read a book aloud together. Strengthening our family bonds daily can be one of the most effective ways to communicate and encourage one another during these unusual times. Let me leave you with the following scripture:

> *"The Lord is my strength and my shield, my heart trusts in Him, and he helps me. My heart leaps for joy, and with my song I praise him."*
>
> —PSALM 28:7 NIV

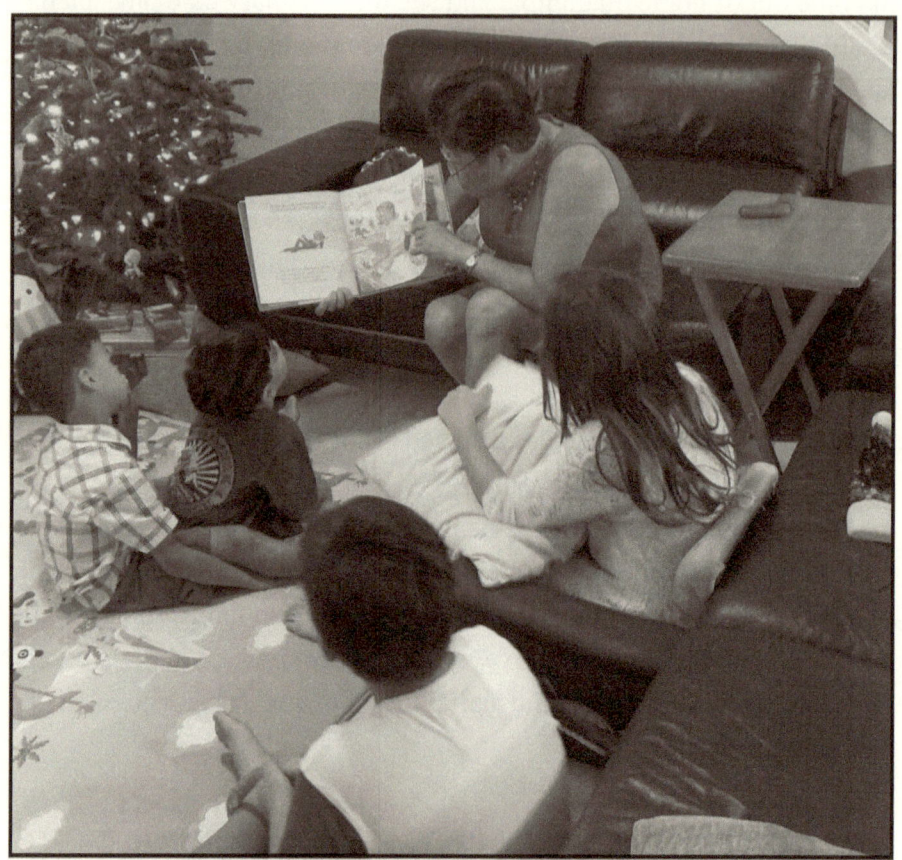

The headlines in our local newspaper yesterday stated that the COVID-19 pandemic may persist for a while. This past week, as I have been seeing some patients for their well-child checkups, many of my families have been telling me how their entire household is in a state of chaos. With our current statewide lockdown, both parents and children are at home and driving each other crazy.

I want everyone to pause and remember that the entire family thrives best when routines and schedules are regular, predictable, and consistent. Many studies have now confirmed what we, as parents and teachers, have long known: that schedules and routines are crucial.

Schedules plan the day by time and activity, and **routines** are how we accomplish the scheduled items.

Schedules build trust within a family, and children know that their needs will be consistently met. When there is a disruption of the routines, anxiety builds, and everyone starts showing emotional reactions to the inconsistencies.

Folks, we're going to be dealing with this pandemic for a while, so let's all have a family meeting and establish an effective routine that everyone can agree on. Here are some tips to help you during these trying times:

Mornings:

- Get things in order the night before.
- Keep morning wake times and routines regular and cheerful.
- Review the day's schoolwork, chores, goals, and other activities.

Afternoon:

- Have lunch together and ensure that all essential "to-dos" have been accomplished.
- Younger children should have their naps, and others have some quiet time.
- For a family activity outdoors or a family project around the house.

Evenings:

- Get the entire family together to prepare for the all-important dinner meal.
- Sit down together and eat without the television or phone.
- Enjoy pleasant family conversations.
- Take some time for family togetherness, such as playing board games, card games, puzzles, or reading aloud together.

Bedtimes

- Stick to regular bedtime schedules.
- Avoid exciting play before bedtime.
- Maintain nighttime rituals as consistently as possible.
- Don't forget to set time aside for yourselves, too.

"The Lord sits enthroned over the food; the Lord is enthroned as King forever. The Lord gives strength to his people; the Lord blesses his people with peace."

—PSALM 29:10–11 NIV

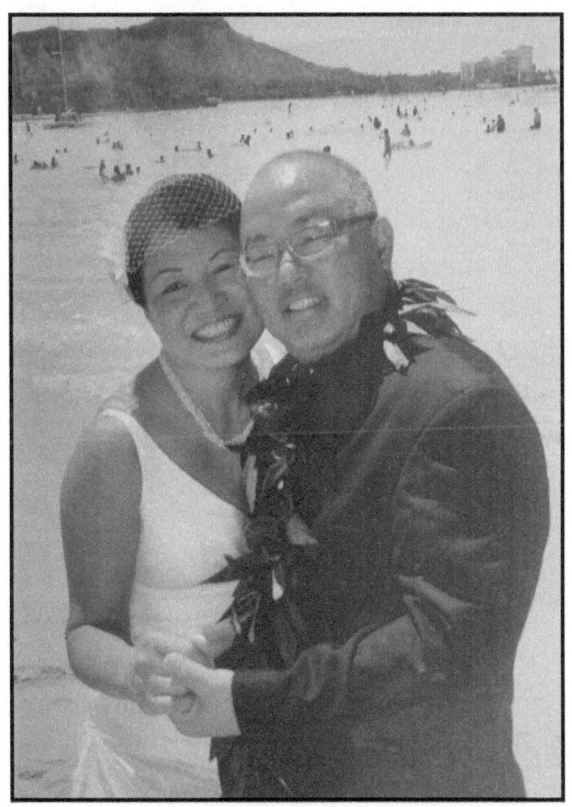

Toady is Saturday, and I awoke feeling sad and frustrated that I had to postpone my weekly Saturday "Walk with A Doc – Oahu" session. We have been meeting at the Patsy T. Mink Central Oahu Regional Park, near the tennis courts, rain or shine, since 2016. Unfortunately, due to lockdowns, we've had to postpone this event for now.

It had been my weekly routine for the past four years, and the walkers have become my second family. I miss the cherished hugs, fellowship, and incredible stories we shared each week.

So, as a substitute, my husband and I decided to walk this on our own. We had a beautiful one-hour morning walk, and it's extra special when you have a partner to do it with. The sun was up, birds were chirping, wonderful trade winds were blowing, and I even ran into a dear friend I had not seen in a while. We had our masks on and kept our social distance while catching up on how we were each doing since the pandemic started.

It's amazing what a little time outdoors in nature can do for you. We are all under a lot of stress and staying at home day after day can start to take its toll over time. Numerous studies have demonstrated that exposure to fresh air enables our brain to absorb more oxygen, which is crucial for maintaining healthy brain function, growth, and recovery. Our brain uses three times more oxygen than our muscles do; therefore, it is susceptible to decreases in oxygen levels. Additionally, spending time outdoors also improves our concentration and reduces stress by producing endorphins, neurotransmitters that help regulate our mood.

In Hawaii, we have no excuse not to be outdoors. Let's make it a priority and give it a try today. I promise you are going to feel so much better, and thank me later for this fantastic tip.

Recently, due to the dramatic slowdown of demand for appointments in the office, I decided to close my office on Saturdays indefinitely for now. With all this free time on hand, I have found myself pausing and reflecting on the many things I have taken for granted.

I am grateful to the people surrounding me, including my husband, Martin, as well as my dear family and friends. Even though I cannot be with them physically, I'm still able to stay in touch with them using the technology available to us. I am grateful for my health and the ability to keep my office open Monday to Friday for our patients and families. I am especially thankful for all the first responders and frontline health-care workers who get up every day, go to work, and risk their health to save others. Most of all, I am grateful for being a part of this great country where fellow citizens are stepping up to help one another.

Locally, I have been hearing many stories of non-profit and faith-based groups stepping up to either volunteer or organize donations to the elderly and others in dire need, to ensure they have their basic needs met. Perhaps this is the silver lining in this worldwide pandemic. Let us all do what we can to conquer this invisible enemy. Each small contribution will bring us closer to wiping out this virus.

> *"Let love and faithfulness never leave you; bind them around your neck, write them on the tablet of your heart. Then you will win favor and a good name in the sight of God and man. Trust in the Lord with all your heart and lean not on your understanding; in all your ways acknowledge him, and he will make your paths straight."*

> —PROVERBS 3:3–6 NIV

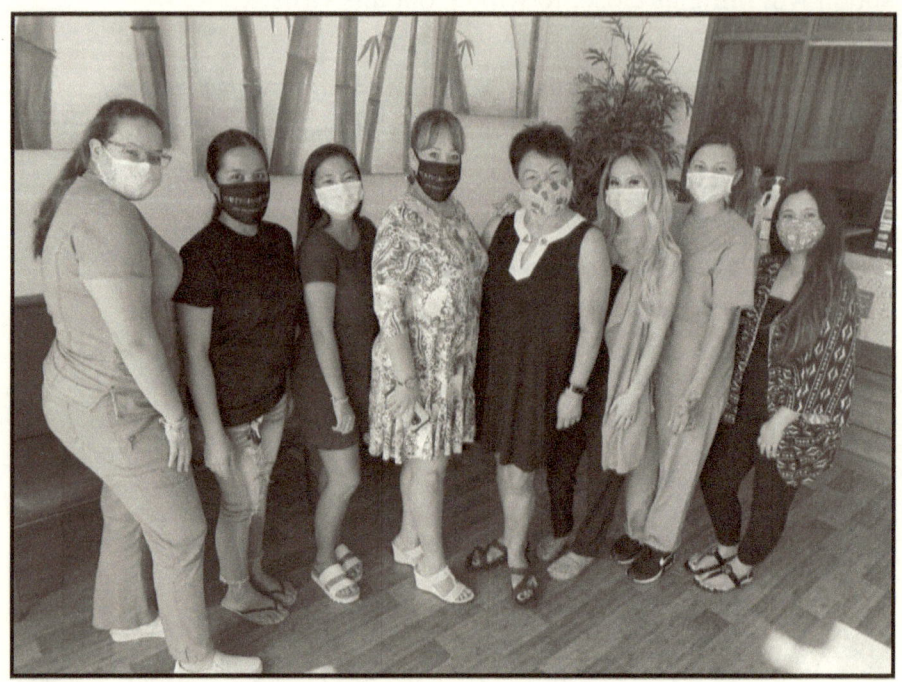

Today, I participated in our first virtual Momilani Christian Church Sunday Service. Due to the shutdowns, we can no longer worship together in person, and this has saddened me greatly. The Sunday worship service was the highlight of my week, and now that it's being held as a virtual Zoom service, it doesn't feel the same. I miss singing and worshipping together, as well as meeting in person with everyone I consider my church family. Somehow, when I'm physically in church, I seem to feel better, forgetting any pain or hardships of the week, and leaving feeling renewed and ready with a spirit-filled soul for whatever the coming week has for me. As it turned out, Pastor Jerry Higashi put together a fantastic virtual service, and it was so comforting to hear his soothing voice and his message. I am deeply grateful for all the effort that went into this virtual production and feel spiritually nourished once again.

Today, we got our daily televised update on the coronavirus. And the numbers appear to be slowly increasing. I anticipate that it will worsen significantly in the coming weeks and months. This all seems like a bad nightmare, but it is our current reality. Let's continue to pray, stay informed, and support one another in these uncertain times.

As a front-line healthcare worker, there is no place for fear. I want to stay positive for my staff, as we go to work each day to care for others. We must be diligent with our hygiene habits to protect ourselves and pray that we avoid contracting the coronavirus. I recently saw a poster which read as follows:

"F.E.A.R. has two meanings: Forget Everything and Run *or* Face Everything *and Rise.*"

> *"So do not fear, for I am with you; do not be dismayed, for I am your God. I will strengthen you and help you; I will uphold you with my righteous hand. All who rage against you will surely be ashamed and disgraced; those who oppose you will be as nothing and perish."*

> —ISAIAH 41:10–11 NIV

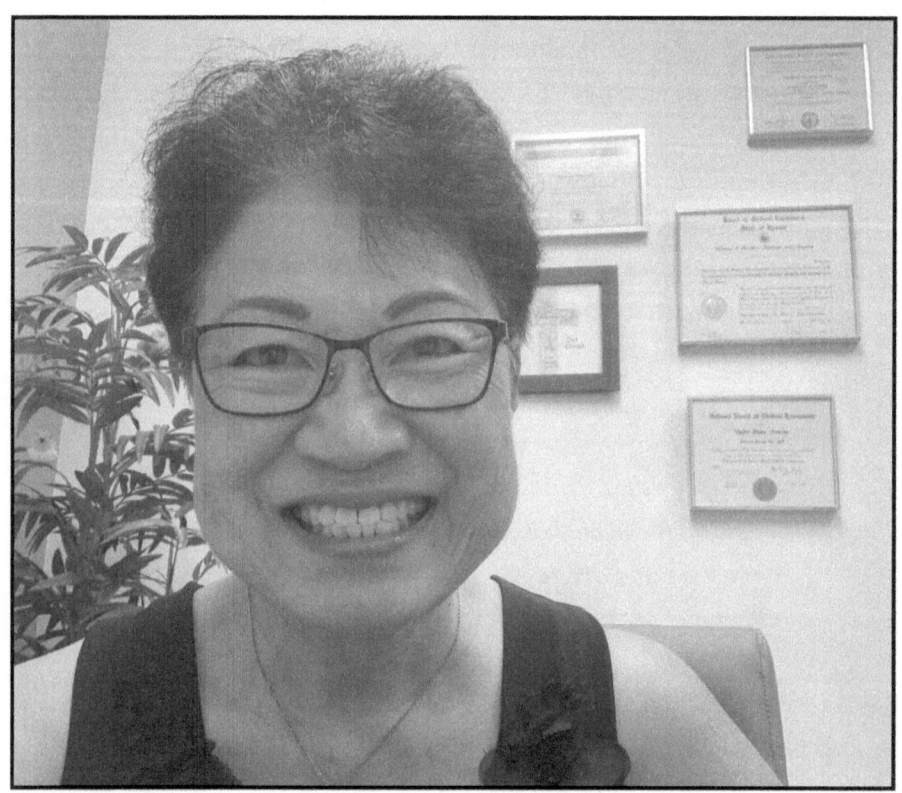

This morning, I dropped fresh flowers off to a few folks I care about dearly. One person I dropped flowers off to asked me what the occasion was, and I told him I was thinking of him. It was an excellent way for me to start the day.

Today is Monday, and I never know what to expect when I walk into the office. Currently, my staff is working to get me set up on the telehealth platform so that I can conduct virtual office visits with my patients online. My associate and I continue to perform our well-child and newborn baby visits, as well as select sick visits, in the office, with meticulous disinfection before and after each visit.

As a small business owner, I face numerous non-medical office issues daily, and I want to stay focused and calm. Some of these issues concern me, such as making payroll, decreasing office hours, ensuring we have sufficient personal protective equipment (PPE) for everyone, and much more, to name a few. The bottom line is keeping myself and my staff safe and healthy, while staying open and providing the best medical care for all our patients and their families.

On another note, did you know that each year, March 30, is National Doctors' Day across our nation? As I listened to Governor Cuomo talk about the COVID-19 situation in New York this morning, I wanted to give a shout-out to those "superheroes," the ER and ICU hospital physicians nationwide, working so hard to keep people alive.

As our leaders and politicians have noted, this pandemic is a war, and our soldiers are all our healthcare workers. However, remember that we have many other unsung heroes, including our food delivery personnel, postal service workers, grocery store workers/cashiers, police officers, EMTs, janitors, bank employees, and many more. Today, let us all be grateful for everyone who comes together and works as a team.

A final reminder for everyone: please do your part by staying at home, washing your hands frequently, and avoiding touching your face. Also, be thankful for your primary care physician, and the next time you see them, take a moment to express your appreciation. I'm certain a kind word will lift their spirits.

> *"Do nothing out of selfish ambition or vain conceit. Rather, in humility, value others above yourselves, not looking to your interests but to each of you to the interests of others. In your relationships with one another, have the same mindset as Jesus Christ."*
>
> —PHILIPPIANS 2:3–5 NIV

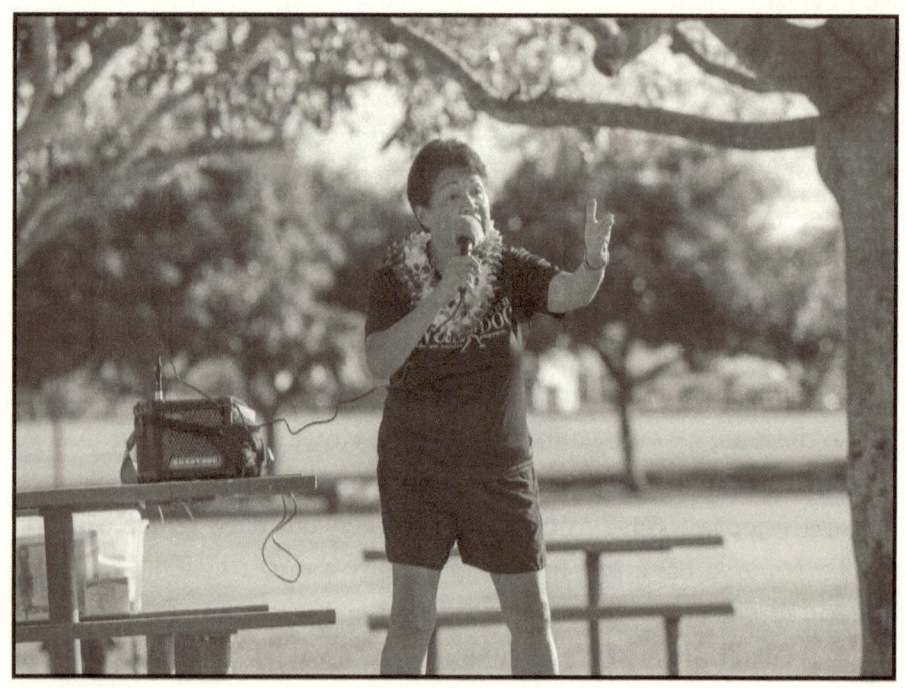

2

APRIL

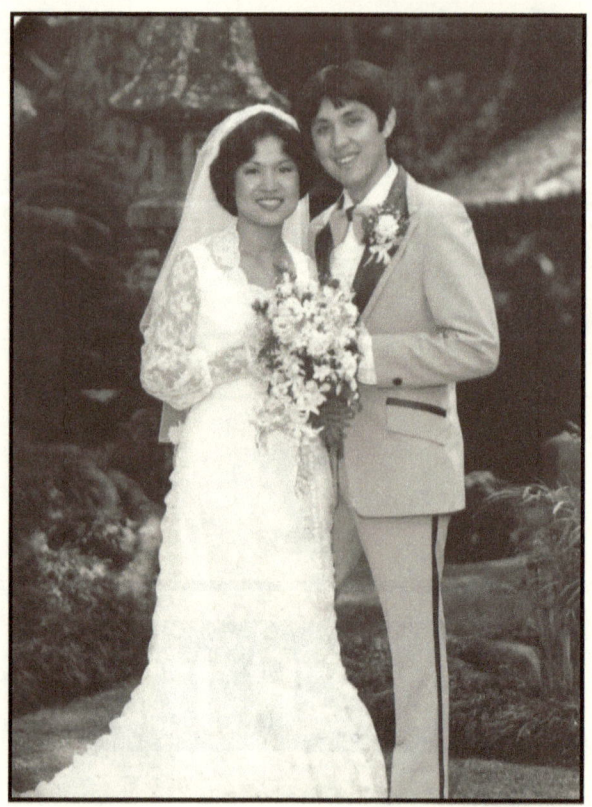

O kay, I'm not going to lie, after listening to the news this morning about the New York situation and how the height of the curve was coming in two or three weeks, I felt despair. How much longer is this going to go on? Today is only April 1, and this is no April Fool's joke. There was even speculation that the pandemic may extend into the summer.

Some questions pop up in my mind: How will we all get through this period on the other side? Are we going to groan or grow? Will we come out more negative or positive? What lessons, if any, would we have learned through this adversity? We have all had adversities in our lives, but we always have the power to choose how we respond to these challenges.

This coming June 11, 2020, will be the tenth anniversary of the sudden and unexpected death of my first husband, Dr. Stephen Wee. He was my husband of thirty years, father of our four children, and my business partner. Stephen and I first met when we were pre-med students at the University of Hawaiʻi at Mānoa in 1972. We had several classes together, and before you knew it, he was giving me rides home in his cute Volkswagen Bug. He was kind and generous, and I always regarded him as a brother. We both got into the University of Hawaii John A. Burns School of Medicine but always remained in the "friend zone" until our final year in medical school.

One evening, he turned to me and said, "I think we should go for it." I was confused and thought he meant to go for ice cream, but I suddenly realized he was talking about getting married. He had always been my best friend and gave me rides home whenever I asked. It made sense to get married, so I said yes, and this was the start of our grand adventure together as a married couple.

We then moved to Columbus, Ohio, for our respective residency training. Stephen did an Internal Medicine Residency at Riverside Methodist Hospital, and I did my Pediatric Residency at Columbus Children's Hospital. We lived in Ohio for six years, and this time alone as a couple, and then as young parents, was a great time of learning to be self-sufficient and mature immensely as a couple.

Stephen and I returned to Hawaii in 1985 to open our private medical practices together in the new community of Gentry Waipio. We bought a modest home, just a few minutes away from the office, and thoroughly enjoyed being a part of this tight-knit community. As time would permit, we both became active in helping with Cub Scouting, Boy Scouts, and the Sabrina Starr Dance Studio, as well as our children's private Christian school, Hanalani Schools. Stephen was also very active as Chief of the Medical Staff for Wahiawa General Hospital, as well as President of the Gentry Waipio Community Association, for many years.

Despite our busy schedules, Stephen and I decided very early in our marriage to have two regularly scheduled dates each week. On our

Wednesday afternoons off, we would have lunch together at the nearby restaurants. We also reserved Saturday evenings as a sacred date night. It was never anything fancy, just a simple dinner and then a movie. I believe these quiet times together helped keep that special spark in our marriage, continuing to grow even stronger each year. Even the children came to regard this as part of their weekly routine and looked forward to spending Saturday nights with their grandparents.

When you think about it, Stephen and I spent our days and nights together, but we somehow never grew tired of each other. We had arguments, like any other couple, but we always knew that they would not last very long.

Friday, June 11, 2010, started like any other day. Stephen and I saw our patients in the office, and at noon, Stephen told me he did not feel well. I immediately told him I would heat our lunch and return. Upon arriving with our lunches, Stephen was unconscious, stiff, and foaming at the mouth. I called 911 and started performing CPR to the best of my ability. The fire department arrived first, and then the EMTs. I quickly called my oldest son, David, that I knew Dad had died.

In that sudden instant, life as I knew it was shattered. With his sudden passing and no forewarning, I was in shock for the first month. It was so hard to understand that he was gone, and I would never see him again. Words could not express the considerable gap that suddenly appeared in my heart. I could not understand how the rest of the world kept moving forward, even though my husband of 30 years had just passed.

I was left with the responsibility of figuring out what to do with his practice as well as my own. I did not even know who I was or what I wanted to do with the rest of my life at 54 years of age. Friends and relatives all had their advice and ideas, but it was all too overwhelming for me to even think about this.

After three months of despair, sadness, and another bout of depression, I got down on my hands and knees one evening and pleaded with God to show me a sign. I was so confused, overwhelmed, and hopeless that I could not even begin to imagine what I wanted to do with the rest of my life.

Within five days, a colleague referred to a job applicant who had 20 years' experience as an office manager. This woman, who lived in my area, was relocating home to Hawaii. I did not even know what an office manager did, but I immediately called and met her as soon as I could.

She was highly qualified for the job and agreed to help my private practice get back on track. She was willing to work for free as a consultant until I was back up and running. However, before we could go any further, she asked if she could say a prayer for me. I stood there in shock and wondered to myself, "Is she the answer to my prayers?"

Since Stephen's sudden and untimely death, my business was on the verge of bankruptcy, but she volunteered her services to help me get my practice up and running. She later told me that I looked so defeated that she felt compelled to pray that God give me the strength to move forward. Through the grace of God and the support of many, I soon bought a new office unit nearby, designed it, and restarted my new practice, Wee Pediatrics, Inc.

It was only through God's grace that I finally accepted this unexpected tragedy and began to focus on taking one day at a time. This was a difficult period, but I know that Stephen would have wanted me to move forward and find happiness surrounded by the love and support of friends. It was only through God's grace that I finally accepted this unexpected tragedy and began to focus on taking one day at a time. This was a difficult period, but I know that Stephen would have wanted me to move forward and find happiness surrounded by the love and support of friends and family.

Yes, I am feeling despair today in this COVID-19 lockdown, but also extreme gratitude for the wonderful group of people who continue to surround me with love. Suffering is a part of life, but we can choose to be resilient and adapt. My advice to you, dear readers, is to spend quality time with your family, as well as quiet time alone, reflecting on all the good in your life. Things will look a little bit brighter. Love is ultimately going to get us through this. Remember, take it one day at a time.

> *"The Spirit himself testifies with our spirit that we are God's children. Now if we are children, then we are heirs – heirs of God and co-heirs with Christ, if indeed we share in his sufferings in order that we may also share in his glory. I consider that our present sufferings are not worth comparing with the glory that will be revealed in us."*
>
> —ROMANS 8:16–18 NIV

ENTRY: 04/02/20

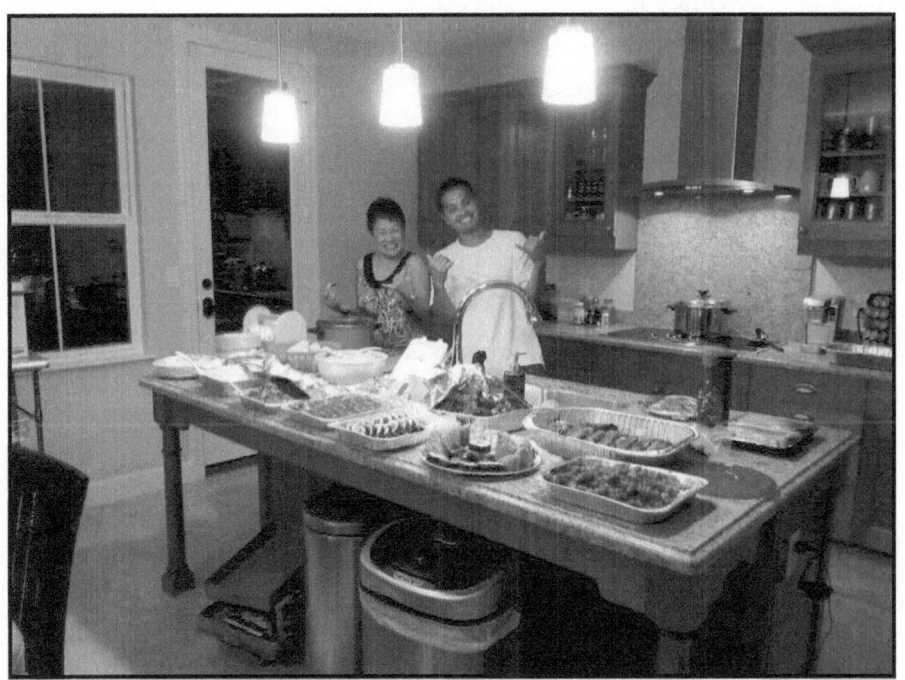

ast night I got a surprise call from my oldest son, David. Our conversations always start with the same greeting, "What are you doing, Mom?" But last night he added one more line, "You feeling okay? Don't die on me." To which I reassured him that I was feeling well.

My oldest son has been a big help to me and my business, Wee Pediatrics, Inc. Ever since my husband passed away ten years ago, he has jumped in without hesitation. He continued to assist me in all aspects of medical practice to keep it alive and thriving. He has also made it a point to stay in touch with his three younger siblings and make sure they are doing well.

He is my unsung hero behind the scenes. I don't pay him a dime, but he spends countless hours managing the books, paying taxes, and assisting my office manager and supervisor nearly every day. In addition to his full-time day job, he is a loving husband and father, cares for his three active boys, cooks, cleans, and does what needs to be done daily. During the COVID-19 pandemic, he has been working tirelessly to ensure my office navigates this current crisis.

His dad and I started our medical practices thirty-five years ago, and he is passionate about ensuring the practice's survival and continued success. Yes, my first son can be extremely grouchy and demanding at times, but he always has my best interests in mind and has a servant's heart of gold. I wanted to pause for a moment and express my gratitude again. I know I've said it a thousand times, but my heart is overflowing with gratitude for the wonderful son you are. At times, I am in awe at what a fine, young man you have grown to be. Dad would have been so proud of you. I know I am!

Tonight, please take a moment to tell someone you love how much they mean to you...

> *"Start children off on the way they should go, and even when they are old, they will not turn from it."*
>
> —PROVERBS 22:6 NIV

ENTRY: 04/03/20

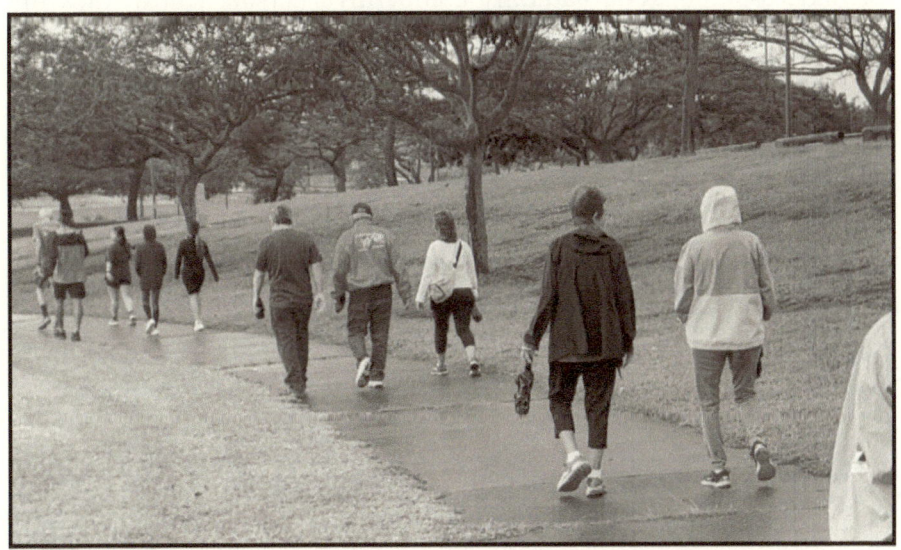

I am proud to announce that my husband, Martin, and I have been very diligent with our evening walks. People seem friendlier than usual, and we always wave to one another. I feel like we are acknowledging that we are in this pandemic together, and we will get through this okay.

So, let's talk about walking.... Walking is the most studied form of exercise that has been proven, time and time again, to improve your health. It is the most popular form of exercise and has one of the lowest injury rates of any exercise. People of all ages can participate in this activity, and it has the lowest rate of injury. Some of the many benefits of walking include lower blood pressure/ cholesterol, lower fasting blood sugar, improved memory, reduced stress, a better mood, and a longer life.

A recent study in the Journal of the American Medical Association (03/20) found that for each additional 4,000 steps someone took in a day, the risk of dying early from heart disease, cancer, or other causes decreased by 50% or more. Additionally, those who achieved 8,000 steps a day fared significantly better and received more benefits than those who achieved 4,000 steps a day or less.

One of the best devices I've ever invested in was a wrist pedometer for under $30.00. As a naturally competitive person, I now track my daily steps and strive to take as many as possible each day. I'm happy to be on a quest to park far away from my destination, so that I can get more steps in after a long day at the office. Whenever I must choose between elevators and stairs, I opt for the latter to challenge myself. For me, movement is essential during my waking hours, and as a result, I am constantly seeking creative ways to increase my activity.

The minimum recommendation for adults is thirty minutes of moderate-intensity walking, five days a week, but more is beneficial. Here are five suggestions to increase the benefits of walking even more:

- Walk as much as you can – something is better than nothing. Ten thousand steps a day is excellent, but take it slowly and gradually; increase your steps as you feel stronger. Pick up the pace – have a shorter walk but do it faster.
- Break it up – take brisk walking breaks of ten minutes, done several times a day.
- Try intervals or "high intensity interval training." Alternate 30–60 second bursts of faster walking with 1–2 minutes of slower-paced recovery.
- Take a walk up a hill. Think of this as a "two for one" special. When you walk up a steep hill, you get the benefits in half the time.

If you have been thinking about taking that first step toward better health, this is your golden opportunity to start.

> *"For we are God's handiwork, created in Christ Jesus to do good works, which God prepared in advance for us to do."*
>
> —EPHESIANS 2:10 NIV

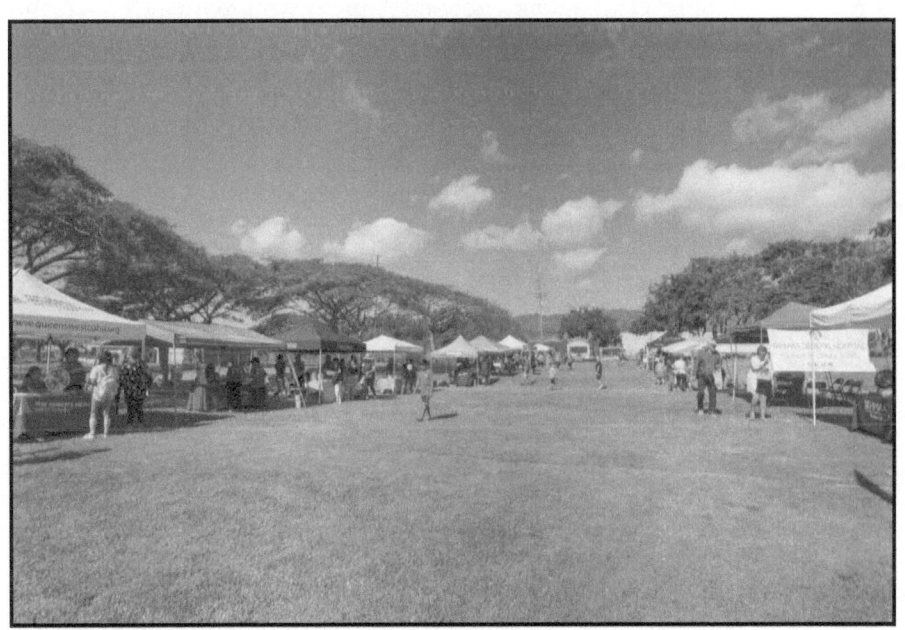

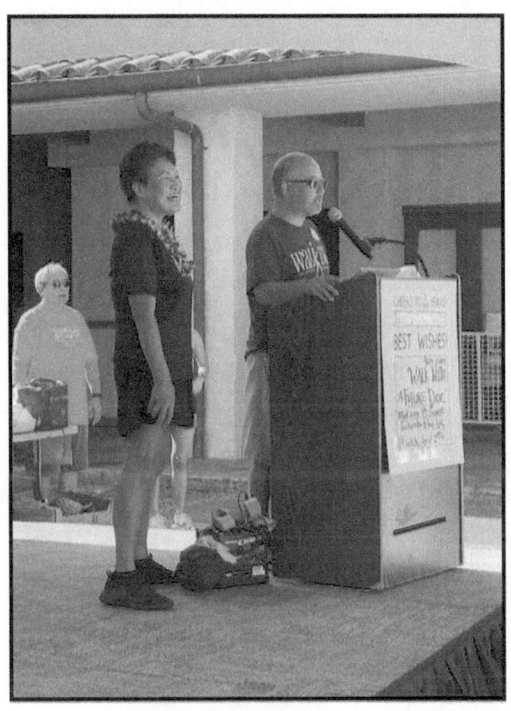

oday would have been a very special day for our "Walk with a Doc – Oahu" Group. Our "Second Annual Walk with a Doc – Oahu Health and Wellness Fair" at Central Oahu Regional Park was set for today, and last year we had over 600 people attend. We had live entertainment and over thirty health vendors participating. My Board of Directors and volunteers started the planning process last year and worked countless hours. However, due to the pandemic, it had to be cancelled for this year.

I am reflecting on how COVID-19 has drastically changed many of our regular annual celebrations and special events. Some personal events that have been cancelled are my mother-in-law's funeral, a friend's wedding, the yearly Hawaiian Island Ministries Conference at the Convention Center, wedding showers, high school graduations, and many more. What I miss the most is face-to-face social contact with my family and friends.

I had a very stressful day at the office today. In addition to seeing patients, I also worked with my staff to complete the application for a forgivable loan, which would provide financial assistance to my business. As I was wrapping up my day and on my fourth and final phone call to a mother, she ended up with words of thanks for my help and told me how much she appreciated me being there for her. This took me by surprise, as people rarely do this. It made this entire week of craziness worth it.

We're surely not the only generation to make sacrifices for the greater good of others. My parents would tell me stories of surviving the bombing of Pearl Harbor and the subsequent days of martial law and food rationing that followed. My grandparents, who immigrated from China, would tell us stories of the sacrifices they made to survive the Great Depression in Hawaii. My maternal grandfather, who was a butcher at Metropolitan Meat Market in Hawaii's Chinatown, would recall days when he would pick up discarded vegetable scraps and cook huge pots of soup for the entire neighborhood to enjoy.

Although the news I watch and listen to daily is depressing, what uplifts me are the emerging stories of love and service to others. This weekend, I plan to do one or two random acts of kindness. You will not only uplift someone's spirits, but yours as well.

"Be kind and compassionate to one another, forgiving each other, just as in Christ God forgave you."

—EPHESIANS 4:32 NIV

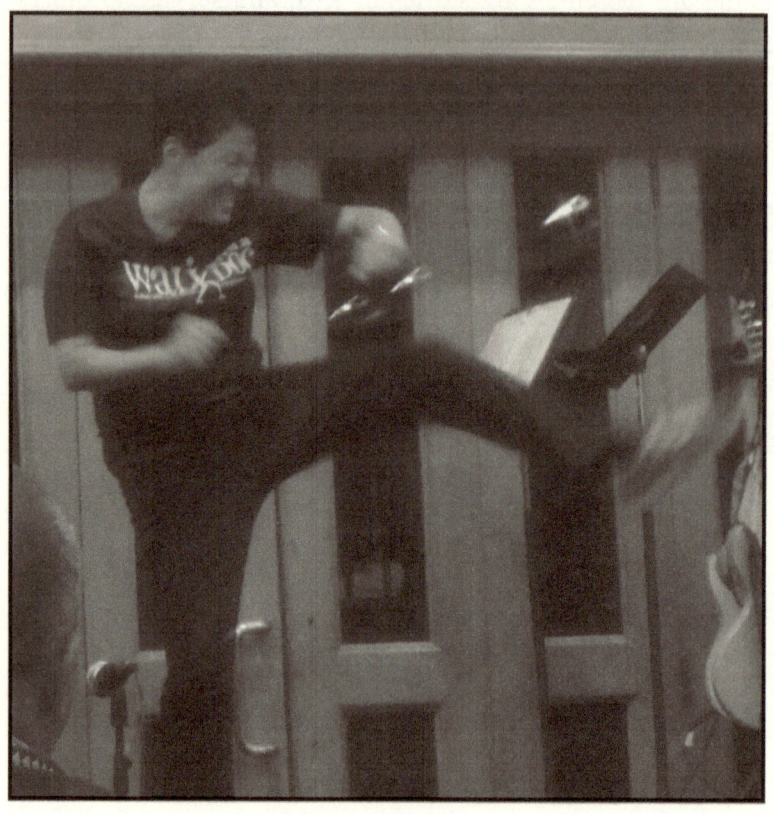

L ast night, I received some bad news. I found out that my dear friend and fellow pediatrician came down with COVID-19.

He is currently in the Intensive Care Unit (ICU) on a ventilator, fighting for his life. This news hit me hard and close to home. Today my heart is heavy. Please include Dr. Lucia Pascua in your prayers as he fights for his life.

I have mixed emotions currently. I sometimes feel like a lamb going to slaughter, being exposed daily to COVID-19, and yet our community needs us to be there. Currently, my associate is on paternity leave, so I am the sole provider in the office for the next several weeks. I will be seeing a full schedule of patients, Monday through Friday, and I can only hope my protective equipment and hygiene habits will keep me safe.

Am I fearful? Yes, I'm not going to lie. I am afraid the virus will get me. During our brief remote church service this morning, my pastor shared a very timely and thought-provoking quote by Mark Twain: "Courage is resistance to fear, mastery of fear – not the absence of fear." I choose today to trust and believe that God is truly in control, and He will care for us. God willing, I will continue to work and only hope that we all do what we are told to do to defeat this invisible enemy.

To my dear friend in the hospital, we are praying for your speedy recovery. We need you; Hawaii needs you. Please don't give up... I know you are a fighter.

Finally, to all my readers, thank you for joining me on this journey over the past two weeks. These are unprecedented times, but through God's grace, I know we will get through this.

> *"For this reason, I remind you to fan into flame the gift of God, which is in you through the laying of my hands. For the Spirit God gave us does not make us timid, but gives us power, love, and self-discipline."*
>
> —2 TIMOTHY 1 6–7 NIV

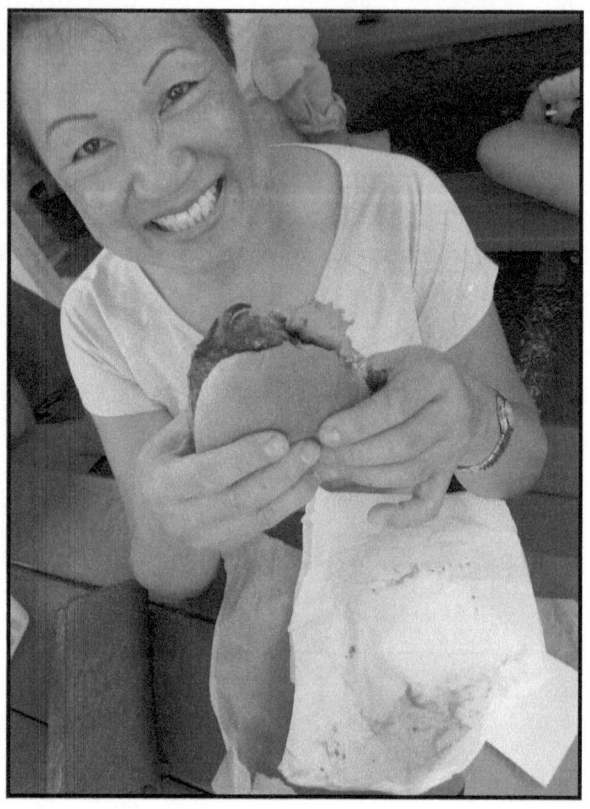

Today was a rough start to the week. I had a very full day of patients at the office and had to wear all my protective gear all day, with only a few breaks. I experienced a lot of sweating and difficulty breathing under all that PPE, but it's necessary for now. I'm learning to live with it, and I'm happy to have an hour-long lunch break midway.

Recently, lunch has become the highlight of my day because it gives me a chance to breathe without a mask, finally get some fresh air, quiet those hunger pangs, and regroup for the afternoon appointments ahead. I have also been taking this time to sit quietly and put down some thoughts for the day, which will help me as I write my blog. I believe that this daily journaling has helped me release some of the pent-up feelings I've been experiencing during this pandemic.

I recently began conducting "telephone call visits" for my patients who are sick. In the past, we always saw our patients in the office; however, during the pandemic, if a patient has a fever or other COVID-19 symptoms, we conduct a telephone call visit. We cannot risk exposing our staff, physicians, or other patients and their families in the office to the virus. The learning curve for these telephone call visits was steep for me, but I think I've finally mastered it. Parents seem very grateful to have the opportunity to speak with me, and I feel fortunate to have the technology to do this. Tomorrow, I'll be jumping onto "FaceTime virtual office visit calls," so wish me luck!

On the news this morning, our nation is expected to face one of the worst weeks of the pandemic. I continue to pray that all the efforts we are putting into "flattening the curve" will help us get through this quicker. I have nothing profound to say tonight, just very physically and mentally drained. I need to get some rest, as I have another full day ahead of me tomorrow.

Special thanks to a good friend who dropped off N95s to my home at 10 PM, as well as another friend who sewed cloth masks for my staff to wear when they are out and about. These little favors and just your encouraging words go such a long way.

> *"The Lord is my rock, my fortress and my deliverer; my God is my rock in whom I take refuge. He is my shield and the horn of my salvation, my stronghold. I called to the Lord, who is worthy of praise, and I have been saved from my enemies."*
>
> —PSALM 18:2–3 NIV

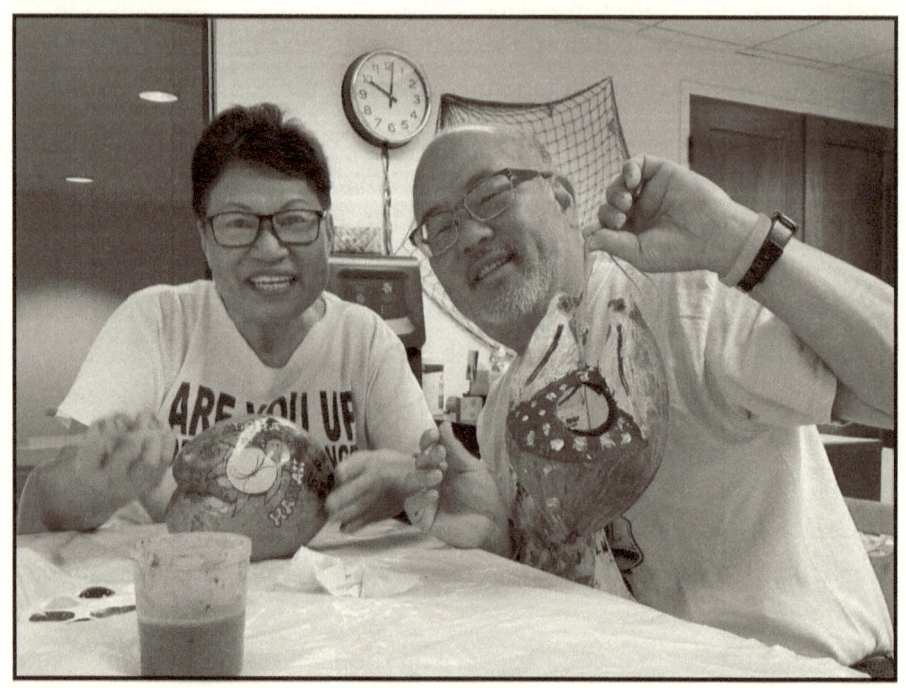

I t's Tuesday morning, and I'm feeling renewed and refreshed after a solid eight hours of sleep. As soon as I turned on the news, the first thing I heard was that New York had its most significant one-day increase of coronavirus deaths – a whopping 731 deaths. Although my daughter, Malia, is currently out of the city, when she returns, this is what she will face.

I made a conscious choice to turn off the news, as I was determined not to let this ruin my day. Just at this moment, a Dunkin' Donuts commercial came on. It was a heartfelt thank you to the many unsung heroes stepping up during this pandemic. They thanked not only healthcare personnel, but also grocery store workers, USPS and other delivery service workers, restaurant owners, police officers, firefighters, maintenance workers, and many others. Everyone has their role during this pandemic, and I'm grateful to everyone who has stepped up and done their job, even in these uncertain times.

I asked Alexa for the definition of "heroes," and she provided the following: A person who is admired or idealized for courage, outstanding achievements, or noble qualities. Today, I truly feel blessed to live in a country surrounded by so many heroes. Just the simple act of caring is heroic, for without this sense of caring, there can be no sense of community.

During these unprecedented times, let us all extend care, kindness, and understanding to one another as we have never done before. We may never know whose lives we touch or improve, but what will be important is that we care and act.

> *"Be kind and compassionate to one another, forgiving each other, just as in Christ God forgave you."*
>
> —EPHESIANS 4:32 NIV

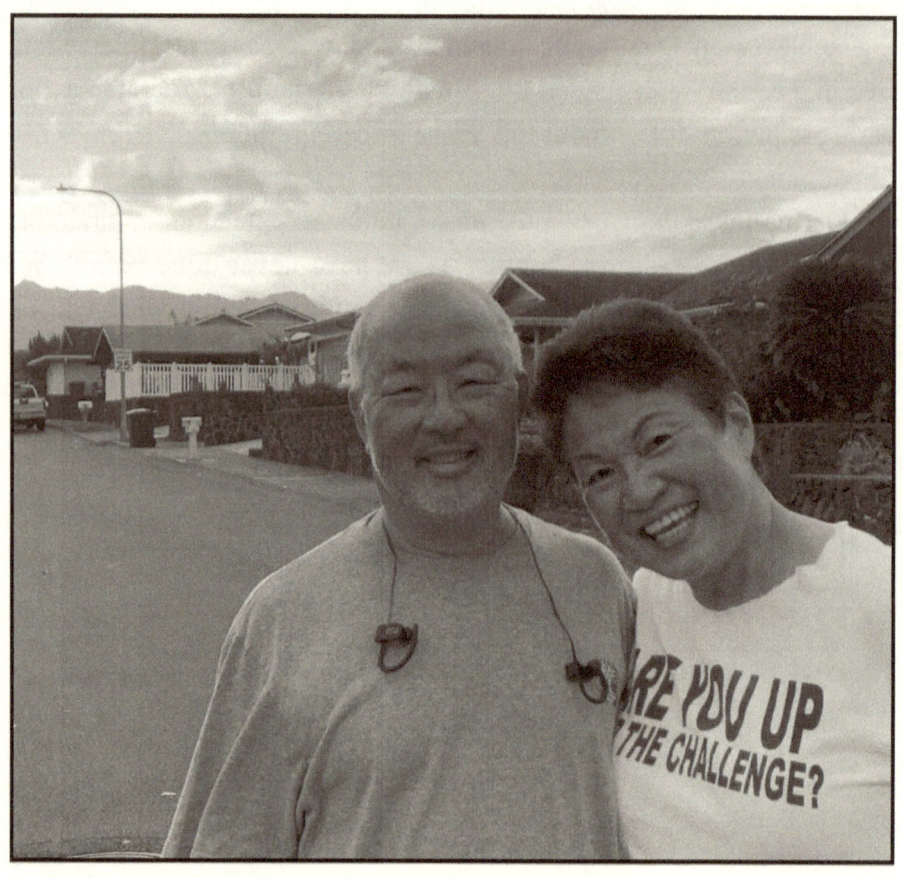

ast night on my walk, I witnessed a beautiful Hawaiian sunset. I stood there in awe and even took a picture of it. We're incredibly fortunate to live in Hawaii. For a moment, I forgot all about the coronavirus and just appreciated this magnificent view. So today, I wanted to share with you some important facts I found out about this essential vitamin – "Vitamin Nature."

Currently, we are all forced to quarantine at home, and if we must go out, we must practice social distancing. Easier said than done…. I don't know about you, but I'm starting to feel a bit of "cabin fever." However, with Hawaii's perfect weather, why not go to your backyard and enjoy the proven benefits of being outdoors?

Studies have shown that taking a brief walk outdoors can significantly improve one's mood, increase energy, reduce stress, and have an immediate positive effect on blood pressure and the immune system. Wow... that's a lot of benefits, and the best part of it is, it's free.

So, let's all get up from our La-Z-Boy chair or office chair and get outdoors for some fresh air. Some suggested activities that might move you into action could be taking your dog out for a walk (he will appreciate it), starting to keep a nature journal, spending time gardening or working outside, or planting a garden at home.

We certainly have the time right now to explore new hobbies or activities, so why not try going outdoors to lift your spirits? I am almost positive you will thank me for it later.

"They speak of the glorious splendor of your majesty – and I will meditate on your wonderful works. They tell of the power of your awesome works – and I will proclaim your great deeds."

—PSALM 145:5–6 NIV

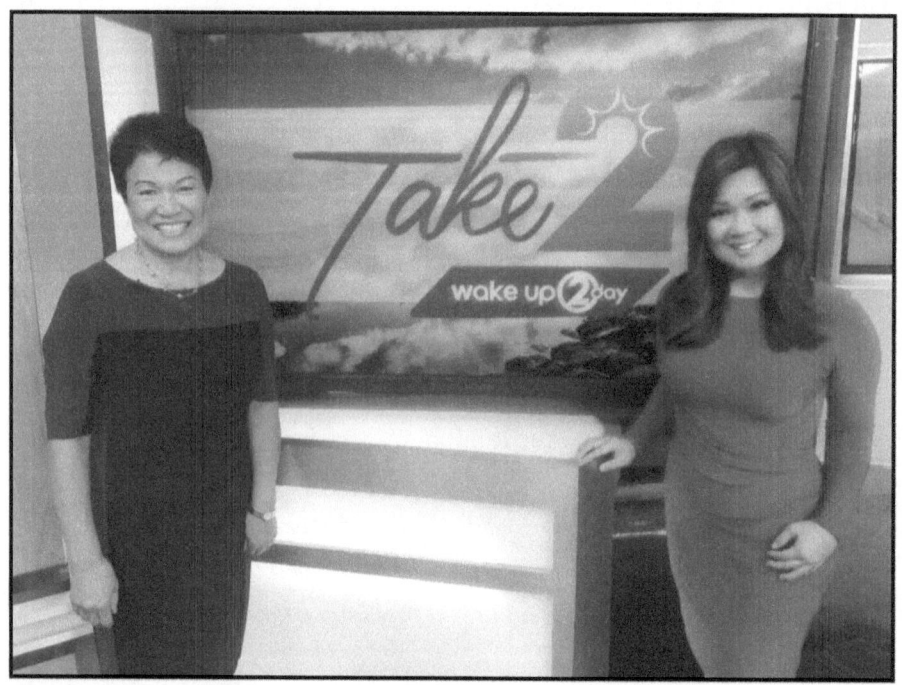

Yesterday, I overheard my five-year-old patient ask her dad, "When is the coronavirus vacation going to be over? I want to go back to school." I suppose that no matter what age we are, we all want things to return to normal. Unfortunately, we are transitioning into a new normal, which will slowly evolve over the next few months or possibly years.

As I worked in the office today, conducting well-baby exams and administering vaccines, I continued to wear my face shield, N95 mask with an overlying surgical mask, and goggles. It seems a little ridiculous and overkill, but I constantly assume that anyone coming to my office, including my staff, could have the coronavirus. My "sick" telephone visits are also a new experience. I can conduct a thorough history and ask questions, but not being able to examine them physically makes me feel that my visit is incomplete. We must do our best under these unique circumstances.

The afternoon was spent discussing the survival of my practice with my management team and ensuring our government loan application was complete and accurate. Every day brings new challenges and changes, and I need to stay on top of everything. I currently have eight employees, and I want to make sure everyone is taken care of as we move forward.

As a medical provider on the front lines, I am feeling the stress and strain from all the uncertainties surrounding me. Will I catch coronavirus today? Do I already have it? Will one of my staff get it? Can I make payroll and rent for the next several weeks? Will my government grant or loan be approved? Will my entire loan be forgiven, or will I owe money back to the government? Am I caring for my patients in the safest and best possible manner? I could go on and on, but you get the idea.

I'll be "live via Zoom" from my office for my monthly Keiki Health Tip on Channel 2's "Take Two Program." I usually attend the studio live, but due to the coronavirus, I will host the show remotely from my office.

This monthly gig has been a blessing for me for the past four years, every second Friday morning. I'm very grateful to have this unique opportunity to educate viewers of all ages on timely health topics. I cannot reiterate this enough: Knowledge is power. And we can all benefit from sound medical advice.

Tomorrow's topic will be on the many benefits of routines and schedules, especially during the COVID-19 lockdowns.

"Dear friend, I pray that you may enjoy good health and that all may go well with you, even as your soul is getting along well."

—3 JOHN 1:2 NIV

ENTRY: 04/11/20

This morning was a typical, beautiful Hawaiian Saturday morning. As I passed by Central Oahu Regional Park on my way to work, I couldn't help but think of my weekly Walk with a Doc – Oahu walking events there for the past four years. Oh, how I miss my Walk Family! I promise you, as soon as this COVID-19 quarantine is over, I will be back there, so don't let your heart be troubled.

As I reminisce about the many lives WWAD – Oahu has touched, I feel so compelled to tell you about the inspirational woman who lit the fire under me to start this walking chapter.

As a twenty-five-year-old UH Medical Student graduate, still relatively inexperienced, I entered one of the most extensive Pediatric Training Programs in 1979, the Columbus Children's Hospital Program (yes, "Buckeye" Country). There were thirty-two other first-year interns, and I was one of only three women in our first-year class. It was not only a cultural shock, but also extremely intense, "on-the-spot" training. On my very first night on call on the Infectious Disease floor, I saw two deaths from bacterial meningitis. The organism causing the death of these two children was the meningococcal bacteria, for which there is now a vaccine that can prevent this horrible disease from killing our children.

This entire first night on call was overwhelming, physically and emotionally. As first-year pediatric interns, we pulled thirty-six-hour shifts every third night, which, of course, is no longer allowed. On the other hand, by spending so much time in the hospital, we gained a wealth of knowledge and insight from these experiences.

During these trying times, I befriended a wise mentor, Dr. Annemarie Sommer, who – for some reason – decided to take me under her wing, like a loving mother. Despite being a world-renowned geneticist, she was extremely humble and showed great compassion to her family. No matter how dire the situation was, she was always able to put her family and patients at ease. I learned many valuable lessons from her, including the essential skills of listening, keen observation, hard work, and perseverance. She always reassured me and seemed to have complete confidence in me, even in those moments when I doubted myself.

Annemarie escaped East Germany as a young woman and came to the U.S. with just the clothes on her back. She initially worked as a janitor, went to a Community College, and eventually worked her way up to attend the Ohio State University Medical School. She was an avid supporter of the Walk with a Doc Organization from the start, fifteen years ago, and had a close friendship with the founder and CEO, Dr. David Sabgir. With her encouragement, I finally started a Walk with a Doc Chapter in Oahu in 2016. We now have two other "Walk with a Doc" groups in our state.

Annemarie and I maintained close contact over the next thirty-five years, until she died in 2018. Thank you, Annemarie, for the lessons you taught me and for being a role model to me throughout my lifetime. I love you and miss you!

> *"Instruct a wise man and he will be wiser still; teach a righteous man and he will add to his learning. The fear of the Lord is the beginning of wisdom, and knowledge of the Holy One is understanding. For through wisdom your days will be many, and years will be added to your life."*

> —PROVERBS 9:9–11 NIV

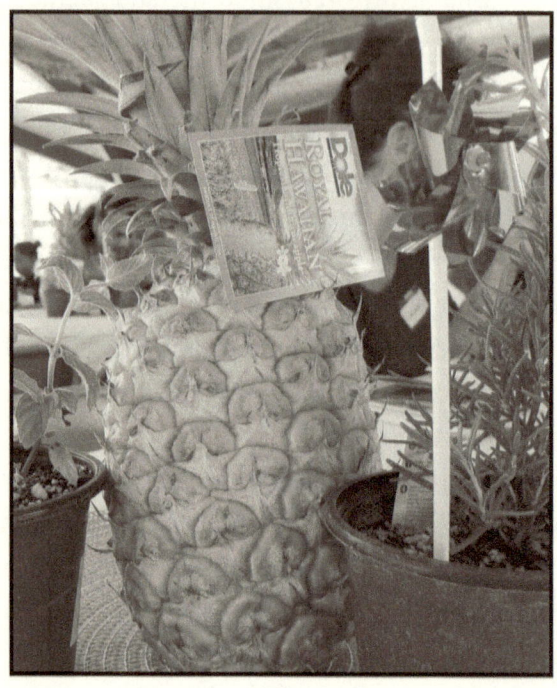

Happy Easter, 2020!

Today, as Christians, we celebrate the resurrection of Jesus Christ from His crucifixion, death, and burial. My husband and I celebrated a quiet Easter at home, listening to several online church services. This has been such a tough time for me, as I dearly miss my church family, especially on this special day.

This past week, there have been unprecedented deaths from the coronavirus, especially in the epicenter of New York. However, there are small glimmers of hope that report we may be reaching the peak and, in some areas, even flattening the curve. The Surgeon General warned us earlier in the week that this may be our "Pearl Harbor" or "9/11" moment, and if we want to get to the other side with the least number of deaths, we all need to do our part.

Yesterday, my husband was kind enough to drive me to Waikiki so that I could get out of the house.

Since I have been in lockdown, my husband took me driving through Waikiki for a change of scenery. The entire area looked like a ghost town until we reached the Cheesecake Factory, where at least fifteen cars were lined up and waiting for their takeout orders. Some things never change.

For the past several weeks before dinner, our prayer has been the same – thanking God for getting us through yet another day of good health as well as healing prayers for all the many lives affected by this deadly coronavirus. In these very unsettling times, there is no choice except to turn to God and trust Him completely.

"Have I not commanded you? Be strong and courageous. Do not be afraid; do not be discouraged, for the Lord your God will be with you wherever you go."

—JOSHUA 1:9 NIV

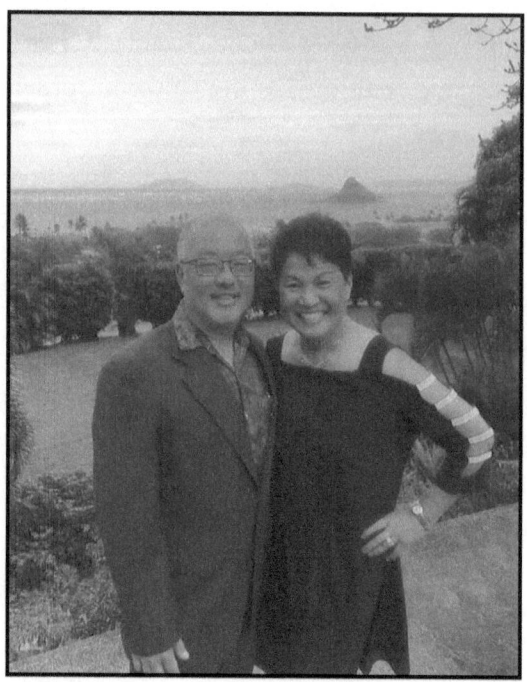

Today, I had the pleasure of seeing many wonderful patients and their families. Many are eager to share stories of how they are adapting to the COVID-19 lockdown. Some people are in better shape than others, but nobody is immune to this pandemic. It's encouraging to hear that families are now sitting down to have meals together, as well as enjoying quality family time and meaningful conversations.

Today, I did seven "tele-health" visits for children who are ill. I'm so proud of myself for accomplishing this technological feat. I never thought I would ever see patients in this way, but it just goes to show that you can teach an old dog new tricks!

As I concluded Holy Week last night, I felt a new peace and perspective I had not felt in a while. I think this change came when I began to pay more attention to what was going on inside me. Ever since the lockdown began, I have been feeling like life was completely spinning out of control, but after some recent reflection, I am now willing to accept and submit to God's plan for my life. I realize I may not see His big plan for me, but I will let God work through me and know that when I bring my concerns to Him, He will give me a peace that surpasses all understanding.

For my physical well-being, I am trying to exercise daily, eat balanced meals, and get sufficient sleep.

What a difference just working on my inner self has made. I am looking forward to a great week and feeling more peaceful and confident. As I close tonight, I urge you to look inward and appreciate the many blessings that surround you daily. When you choose to focus on the positive aspects of your life, your mind, body, and spirit will experience peace and harmony.

"May the God who gives endurance and encouragement give you the same attitude of mind toward each other that Christ Jesus had, so that with one mind and one voice you may glorify the God and Father of our Lord Jesus Christ."

—ROMANS 15:5–6 NIV

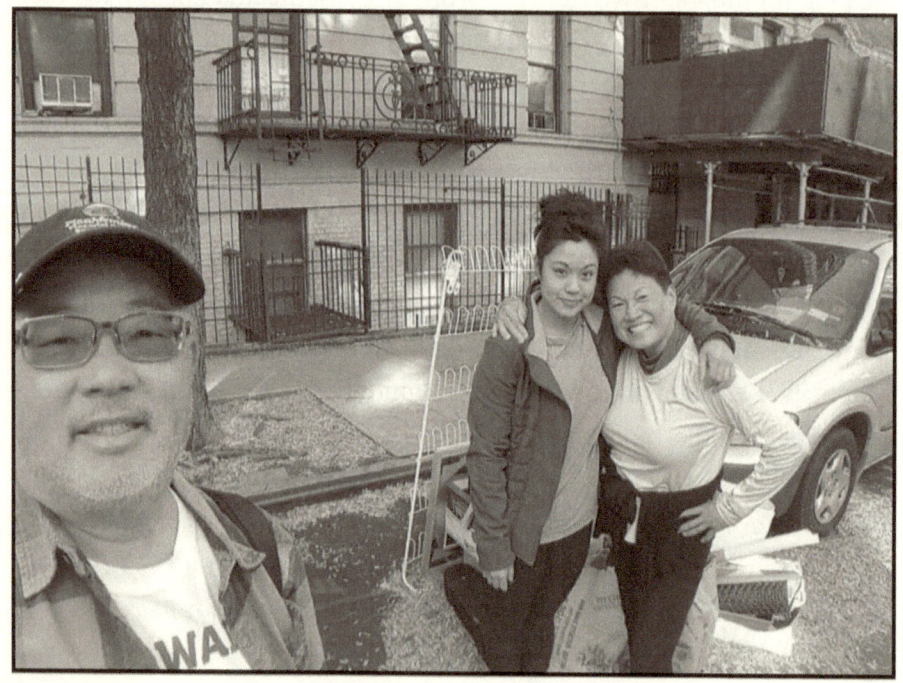

couldn't wait to share the fantastic news about my dear friend and fellow pediatrician, Dr. Lucio Pascua, who came down with COVID-19 and was fighting for his life in the ICU. I spoke of his plight in Entry of 04/05/20, and he is now off the ventilator and expected to make a full recovery. I am deeply grateful for the prayers you sent his way.

This COVID-19 pandemic has radically changed the way we practice medicine. Telephone visits and virtual tele-health visits are now commonplace in the future of medicine. I now see that change is inevitable during this pandemic, and we all have a choice to fight it or embrace it. For myself, I am trying my best to adapt, learn from others, and stay positive. I'm fortunate to have the right people around me to help me through this challenging time. I am not perfect and continue to make mistakes, but I'm learning so much about my business, technology, and new ways of practicing medicine.

Perhaps this is the silver lining of this pandemic.

I received an uplifting, though belated, homemade Easter greeting card from my youngest child, Malia, who resides in New York. We now Skype often, but receiving "snail mail," holding it in my hands, and re-reading her letter of love and encouragement meant so much to me.

So, I had this idea to share with you, my readers. Take a few minutes to sit down and write a letter or card to a friend or loved one, especially if they are living alone. I know it will mean a great deal to them to receive a surprise letter or card.

"Therefore, encourage one another and build each other up, just as you are doing."

—1 THESSALONIANS 5:11 NIV

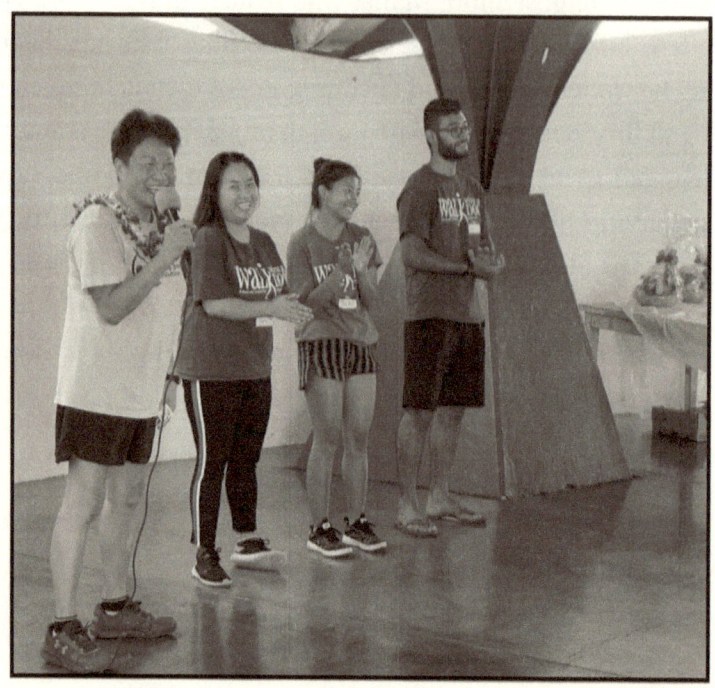

Last night, my husband asked me, "So how long are you planning on doing these blogs?" I told him that I was determined to do these until the end of April. For the most part, it has proven to be a worthwhile endeavor. I have now made it a habit to review my day, open my eyes to my feelings, and see the good in my life. As I sit down to write my blog, I take an inventory of my day and, to my surprise, discover those little blessings that are buried deep within.

I am currently listening to an audiobook, "The 360 Degree Leader," in my car by one of my favorite authors. His name is John Maxwell, and he recently did a podcast because he felt that there was a significant deficit of hope during these dark and unprecedented times. He shared three questions that he thought we should be asking ourselves every day during this COVID-19 crisis:

- How can I use this to improve?

- How will I use this to help others?
- What action will I take to improve my situation?

Spending just a few minutes daily to pause and reflect on these questions can help make ourselves and the world a little better. He goes on to say that we all have good intentions or desires, but we need to step out of our comfort zone, bridge the gap, and act. This is the perfect time to act on our life's purpose and ensure we have no regrets at the end of our lives.

Are you sitting on the sidelines of life, watching the game, or are you actively participating in the game of life to make a difference? It is only by doing that we can make a difference in other people's lives. Leave your legacy for years to come by pursuing a unique mission that only you can accomplish, benefiting others.

I love this quote by Ralph Waldo Emerson: "The purpose of life is not to be happy. It is to be useful, to be honorable, to be compassionate, to have it make some difference that you have lived and lived well."

"In him we were also chosen, having been predestined according to the plan of him who works out everything in conformity with the purpose of his will, so that we, who were the first to put our hope in Christ, might be for the praise of his glory."

—EPHESIANS 1:11–12 NIV

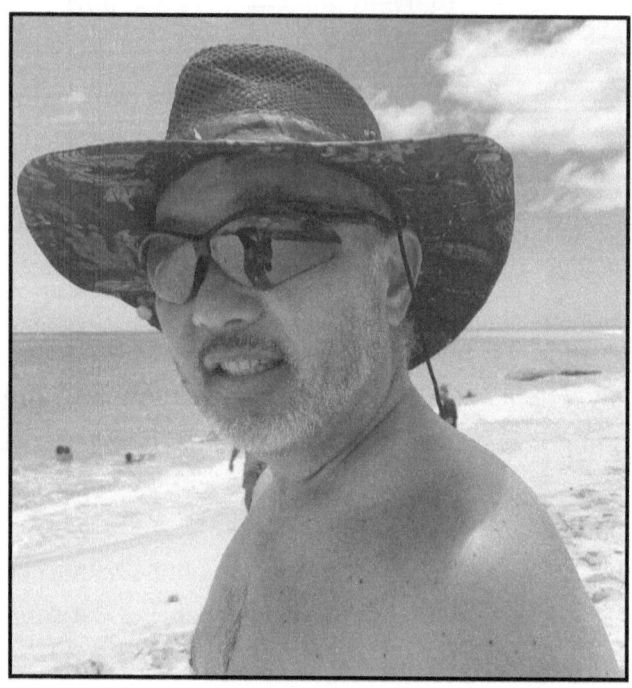

Today, I want to give a loving shout-out to my husband, Martin M. Arinaga. If you've been following my story, you know that Martin is my second husband. I lost my first husband, Stephen, in a tragic instant ten years ago. His death left an enormous void not only for our family but also for our community.

For myself, losing my spouse was so earth-shattering and life changing. It felt like half of me was "torn away," and I wondered if I would ever be happy again. I've had so many ups and downs, just like all of you. The one lesson I have learned through all of this is that life is precious and unpredictable. I now wake up each morning with joy and a feeling of urgency to do as much as I can for the time I have left here. I feel God has allowed me a second chance, and I'm going to make the best of it.

As I go through this COVID-19 pandemic, there are so many uncertainties, but the one certainty that I hold onto tightly is God's love for me and every one of you.

I am off to donate blood today, and I encourage each of you to consider doing the same.

> *"I will say of the Lord, 'He is my refuge and my fortress, my God, in whom I trust.' Surely, he will save you from the fowler's snare and from the deadly pestilence."*
>
> —PSALM 91:2–3 NIV

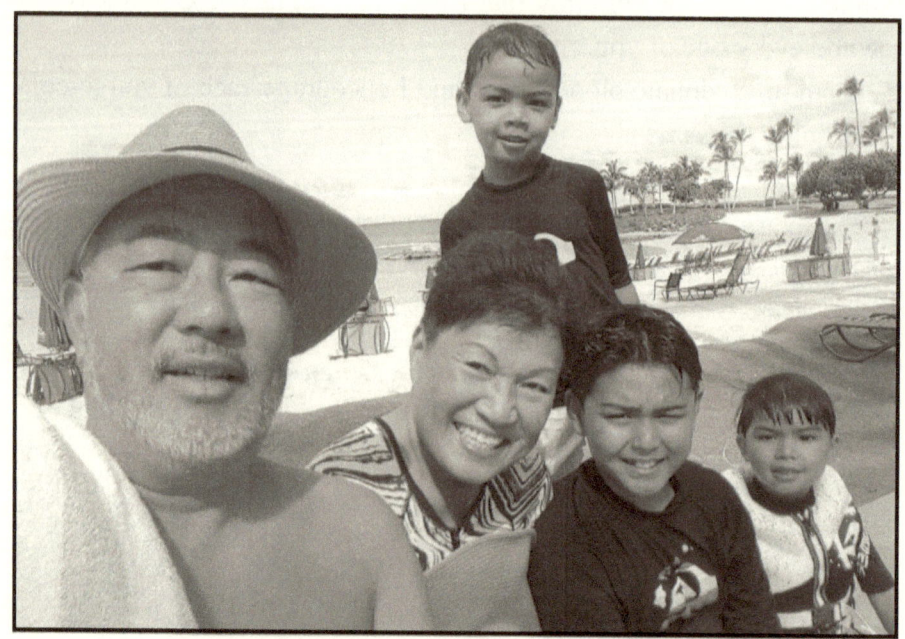

During this COVID-19 pandemic, our lives seem so predictable. Sometimes I forget what day it is. There are no special dinners, celebrations, or other special events on our calendar. The highlight of my day was our early evening walks around the neighborhood. Sometimes, I feel like I move through my daily life like a robot, never pausing to reflect and ask some hard questions, such as who I am or what my life purpose is.

A few months after Stephen's death, my office manager asked me a question which no one had ever asked me before: "What is your passion?" I had been so busy, working in the office six days a week and raising four children, that I never stopped or even ventured into this uncharted territory. I immediately answered that my passion has always been to help my families, especially those struggling with obesity, become healthier. As a working mother myself, I knew intimately the struggles of the working parent and felt that I now have some wisdom, empathy, and experience to help others.

This was my "a-ha" moment, and I knew I had to tackle this. With the help and encouragement of my new practice manager, I immediately began conducting family obesity workshops for families who were ready for change and sought assistance. I recruited volunteers from my community to assist me, and these workshops were a huge success. The initial groups I worked with began showing excellent results. However, after a year, these workshops were held due to the enormous amount of money and time constraints.

I felt my community still needed a nearby program open to everyone that would encourage a healthy lifestyle. In February 2016, my non-profit organization, "Walk with a Doc – Oahu," began. What makes this such a fantastic event is not only the walking we do together weekly, but the new health tips I share, the camaraderie, and, most of all, the friendships we have formed over the years. Nearly every week, I would have walkers come to me in tears, thanking me and telling me what a difference this had made in their lives.

The reality is, I am the one who is blessed. The satisfaction and love that emanate from doing this are indescribable, and I have never been happier. My life is incredibly fulfilling, and I am certain that this is my true purpose in life. There is so much more for me to do, so I will continue to pursue it with urgency each day.

I hope you will pause and *not* wait for a tragedy to happen before you realize your life's purpose. Please make a difference now and don't wait until it is too late.

> *"And we know that in all things God works for the good of those who love him, who have been called according to his purpose."*
>
> —ROMANS 8:28 NIV

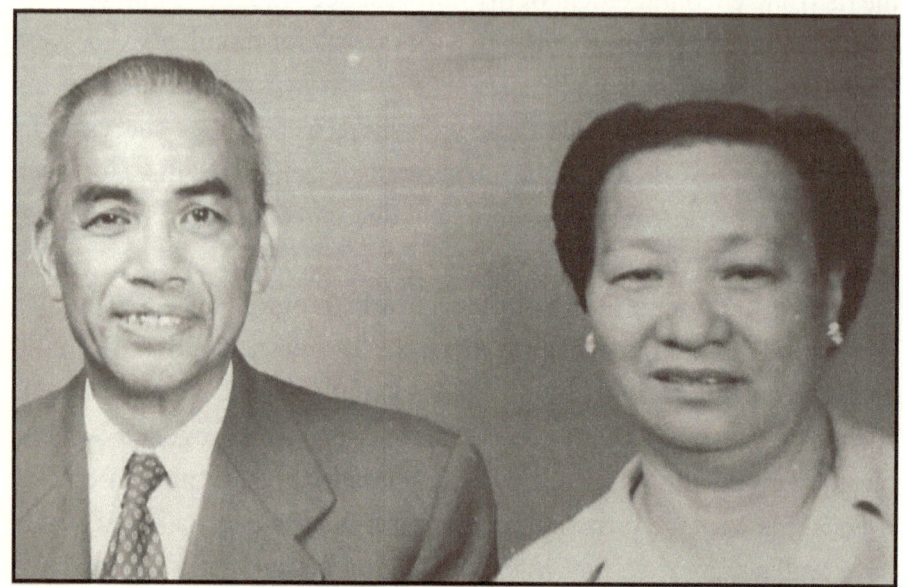

Today was a glorious Sunday… I slept in till just after eight – very unusual for me. I got a surprise call from Malia, which always worries me a little. She remains in Pennsylvania and says she just called to check on how I'm doing. I miss her, but just hearing her voice made my day start great. She told me that she has been doing a lot of reading recently.

She is currently reading *The Good Earth* by Pearl S. Buck and has started asking me questions about her great-grandparents from China. My maternal grandparents lived with us when I was growing up, and they always loved to tell the same old stories, again, about the good old days. I wish I had paid better attention to them.

My grandfather, born in 1899, came to Hawaii as a young boy and only had an elementary school education. He wore a pigtail throughout his teenage years and told me stories about old Hawaii, and how Waikiki was just a big swampy duck pond. He married my grandmother, who was sent over as a picture bride. The rumor was that she ran away when it was time to bind her feet in China. As a result, my grandmother, who had large feet, was considered unmarriageable and not suitable for marriage in China. My maternal grandparents successfully assimilated into American society and raised four children.

I admire my daughter's interest in her past and feel it is essential to understand our roots. I often think about the many sacrifices that previous generations have had to make in this new country. Every generation has had its crises to deal with, but that's just a part of life. The coronavirus pandemic is just one of the many challenges we are currently facing, and I know we will face more in the future.

To my dear readers, thank you for continuing to read my blogs during this unprecedented time. Even though we can't be physically together, just seeing your "likes" or short comments makes me happy to know we are connecting. Although COVID-19 is forcing us into social isolation, I'm comforted by the fact that we can still connect to friends and family via technology. In these times of crisis, reaching out to others in a positive way to reduce loneliness can benefit our health simply by fostering connections. Together, we will all get through this.

I will reach out to my three sons and daughter this afternoon. Why don't you surprise someone with a FaceTime call?

"Do nothing out of selfish ambition or vain conceit. Rather, in humility value others above yourself, not looking to your *interests but each of you to the interests of the others.*"

—PHILIPPIANS 2 3–4 NIV

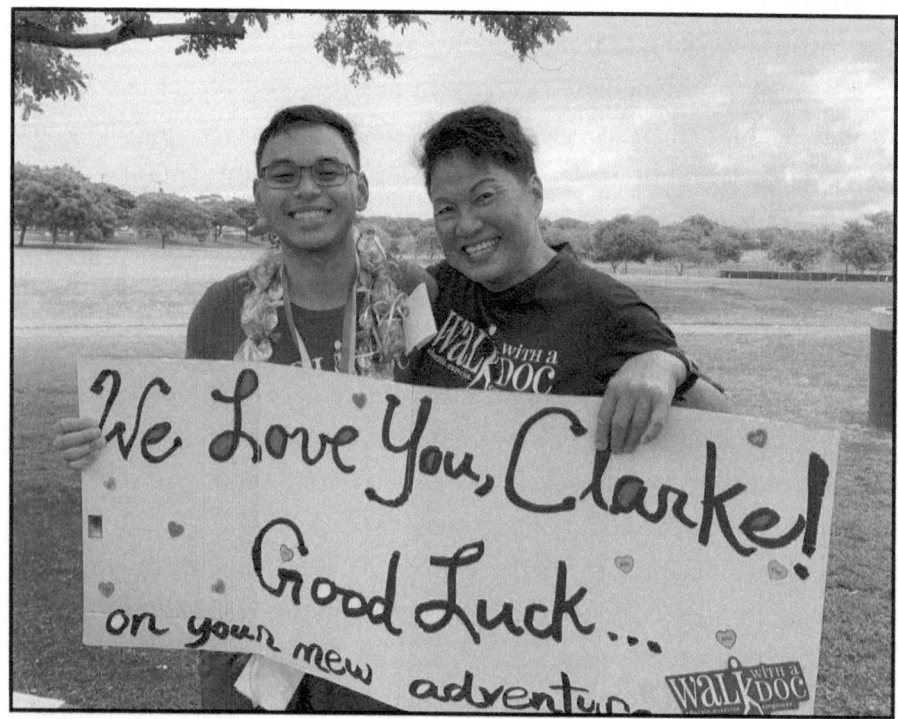

ecently, several parents have told me that their child's well-office visit was the highlight of their week. For many families, this was the first time they had ventured out of the house in weeks. These are trying times for everyone, but as one of my parents told me, "I was given lemons, so I am making lemonade."

I pondered this thought and realized we all have a choice on how we weather the rest of this coronavirus pandemic. We truly have the power to choose our thoughts, words, and attitudes, so why not make it hopeful? As we all adapt to changes daily, let us all keep hope stirring within us.

In my 04/01/20 entry, I mentioned that the tragic loss of my husband ten years ago shattered me into a million pieces. I could have chosen to give up, but instead, I decided to continue forward, despite the fear and uncertainty. The worst had already happened to me, and I was curious about the possibilities that lay ahead for me.

According to the Merriam-Webster Dictionary, the definition of hope is: "(noun) A desire accompanied by expectation of or belief in fulfillment."

I believe that having hope comes down to having a positive mind-set. The best way to do this is to refuse the negative and instead look forward to the victory around the corner. Hope is the anchor of our soul. In turbulent times, our minds and emotions will remain steadier if we are anchored. This storm will not last forever, and we can all learn something from our experience. My prayer for all of you is that you hold onto hope and know that something good will come out of these challenging times.

Today, I got a surprise visit from one of my favorite medical students, Clarke Morihara. He dropped by my office to say hello and left gifts for my office staff, including gloves and N95 Masks. I cannot tell you how happy I was to see him. You see, Clarke shadowed me in the office and then worked part-time for me for about two years. He faithfully showed up every Saturday morning to assist me with my "Walk with a Doc – Oahu" weekly walks. He is now completing his first year of medical school, and anyone who has gotten to know him knows what a great physician he will become.

Thank you, Clarke, not only for your gifts and surprise visit today, but for allowing me the honor of being your mentor! Congratulations on completing your first year of medical school and for giving me great hope for our future physicians.

> *"May the God of hope fill you with all joy and peace as you trust him, so that you may overflow with hope by the power of the Holy Spirit."*
>
> —ROMANS 15:13 NIV

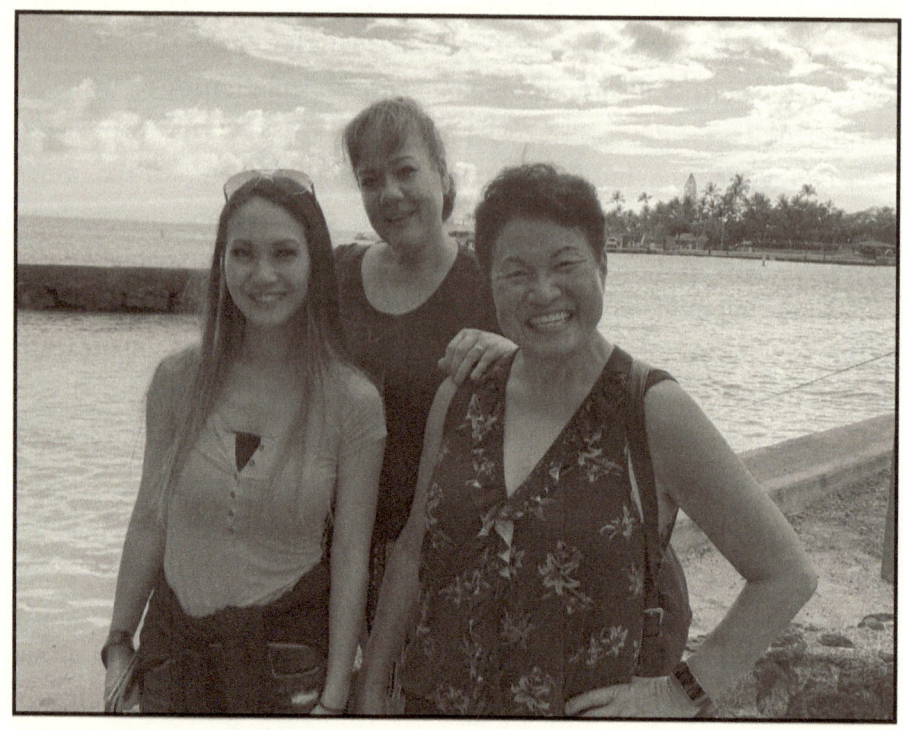

Nearly every morning when I arrive at my office, I try to have a quick huddle with my staff for the "morning briefing." With the ongoing pandemic, there have been daily adjustments in various areas, including scheduling, office hours, and bank loans, among others.

Through all this craziness, I am realizing how fortunate I am to have such a dedicated and loyal staff. Everyone has been flexible and has readily adapted to the ongoing changes. Having such a great team on board is priceless; money cannot buy this type of dedication and care for our patients, families, and each other.

A big shout-out to Danielle, my practice manager, and Kristen, my clinical supervisor, who have been working tirelessly alongside me. Last night, the news reported that many small medical practices will not survive, but I know with certainty that Wee Pediatrics, Inc., will.

For the past three weeks, I have been seeing patients in the office daily, as my pediatric associate has been on paternity leave. It has been a hectic time, but I was told today that, although I may complain about the many new changes, such as telehealth visits, I will eventually adapt to and master them. That was such a nice compliment, and I hope I will always be willing to make the necessary changes that ultimately benefit the practice.

So, perhaps this is what I am learning through all of this: that I can adjust with the support of a great team.

Thank you, Danielle and Kristen, for all you have done and continue to do daily for the practice. A big thank you to my entire staff as well for showing up to serve our community. Excellent teamwork, everyone!

T.E.A.M.

- Together
- Everyone
- Achieves
- More

"Each of you should use whatever gift you have received to serve others, as faithful stewards of God's grace in its various forms. If anyone speaks, they should so as one who speaks the very words of God. If anyone serves, they should do so with the strength God provides, so that in all things God may be praised through Jesus Christ. To Him be glory and power for ever and ever. Amen."

—1 PETER 4:10–11 NIV

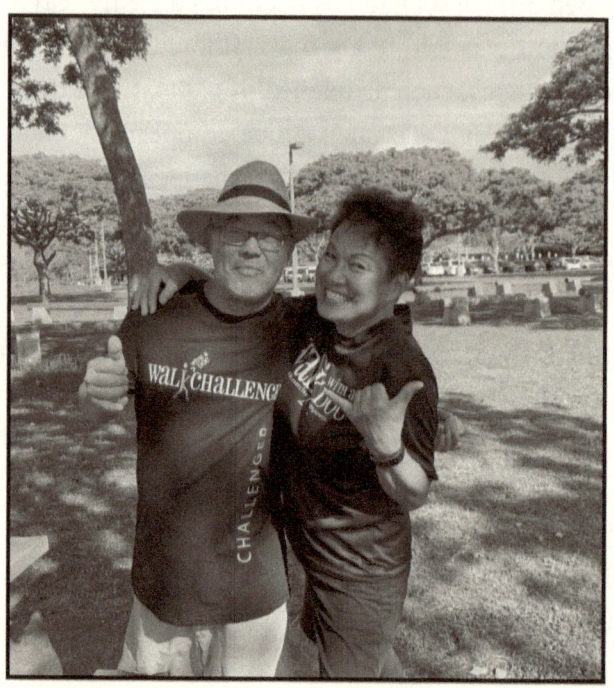

Last night, when I heard that the "stay-at-home" order on Oahu will be extended for one more month to May 31, I got such a sinking feeling in my stomach. Seriously, another month of this... I feel like I can barely make it to the end of April. I'm sure I'm not the only one who feels this way. I immediately realized how easy it was for me to get discouraged, depressed, and cynical about this entire pandemic situation.

This made me think about how we must be cautious about our thinking. It is so easy to fall into those negative thoughts, but these only bring us down and defeat us. Looking at the positives, however, will lighten and lift us.

When I was in high school, the required reading was *The Diary of Anne Frank*. These were the memoirs of a teenager whose family secretly hid in a 450-square-foot attic room for 790 days. During a trip to Europe many years ago, I even got to visit this historic site and recall how small this living space was. In her book, she describes the ways she survived these times, and one of the most important ways she did so was by purposefully finding things, no matter how small, to be thankful for. Our situation is nothing like what she faced, but we can learn a lot from Anne Frank's memoirs. Things are not as bad as they could be, and we can always find something to be thankful for every day. I am here to encourage you to place your trust in God.

Use this time at home wisely by getting plenty of rest – watch uplifting movies, play family board games, read a good book out loud as a family, work on projects you've been postponing – just don't let yourself get bored. Remember, fear is knocking on all our doors, but we need to take courage and walk into this fear with faith to conquer it. I will leave you today with these comforting words:

> *"The Lord is my shepherd, I lack nothing. He makes me lie down in green pastures, he leads me beside quiet waters, he refreshes my soul. He guides me along the right paths for his name's sake. Even though I walk through the darkest valley, I will fear no evil. For you are with me; your rod and your staff, they comfort me."*

> —PSALM 23:1–4 NIV

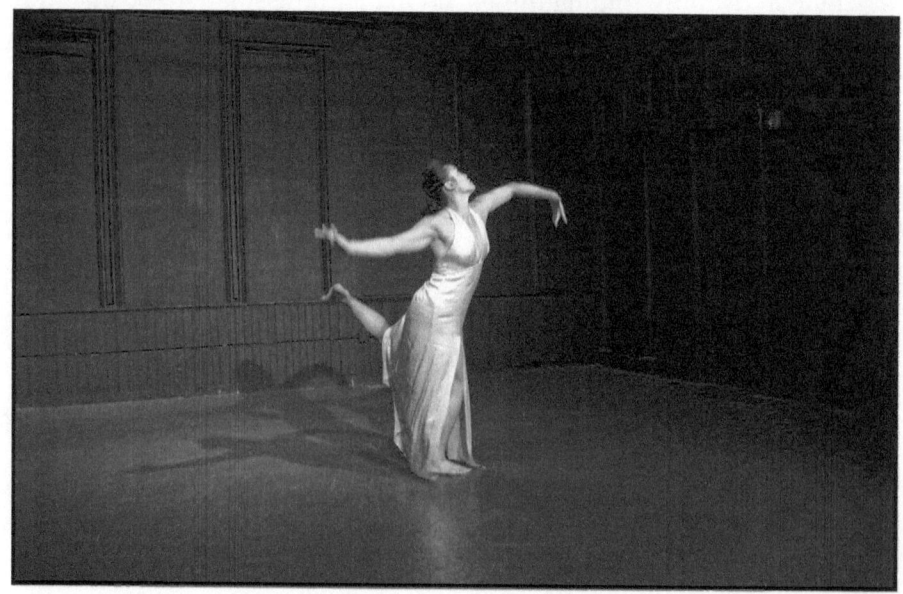

Today is my youngest child's birthday, Stephanie Malia Wee. Due to the COVID-19 pandemic, I was unable to visit her in New York this year. However, to improvise, she invited me to the most awesome "Coronavirus Quarantine Zoom Video Dance Birthday Party," with her and her friends, from across the nation. We all got to meet each other virtually, learn and perform two dances for her, and even sing Happy Birthday to her. As my daughter would say, "great mems." (For those of you not keeping up with the latest, "mems" means "memories.")

Thirty-one years ago, God blessed our family with a daughter, Stephanie Malia Wee. We already had three active Wee boys, but Stephen and I decided to have one more child to complete our family.

Growing up with three older brothers made her "tough as nails. She was an honorary member of our Cub Scout Pack and excelled in climbing light poles, running races, and shooting BB guns.

By the tender age of five, she had become quite independent in preparing for dance recitals, parades, and other performances on her own. She continued to pursue her love of dance while in high school, excelled in musical theater and sports, as well as her academic studies. Her brothers were always tough on her during sports practice sessions and made sure she upheld the "Wee reputation" in school athletics.

The one thing I admire the most about her is her grit and determination to follow her heart. She had told Dad and me, a year before his death, that she wanted to give New York a try after graduating from Westmont College. She kept that promise to Dad and me, packed a suitcase, and bought a one-way ticket to New York City. My little girl has lived in New York City for the past nine years. She is a survivor and has made it on her own. She initially worked in various jobs over the years, which allowed her to pursue her passion for taking lessons in modern ballet and modern dance, choreographing, volunteering at nonprofit organizations, and even producing a few of her original shows.

Malia's grit and determination are excellent examples for all of us right now during this COVID-19 pandemic. She keeps rolling with the punches and always seems to get back on her feet. She is not afraid to pursue her dreams, no matter what the circumstances look like around her. Malia, I am so proud to call you, my daughter. I know Popsie would agree and is looking down at you today with a great big smile! Sending our love and birthday hugs to you today. Love you, Sis. Stay safe. Mama

"It gave me great joy when some believers came and testified about your faithfulness to the truth, telling how you continue to walk in it. I have no greater joy than to hear that my children are walking in the truth."

—3 JOHN 1:3–4 NIV

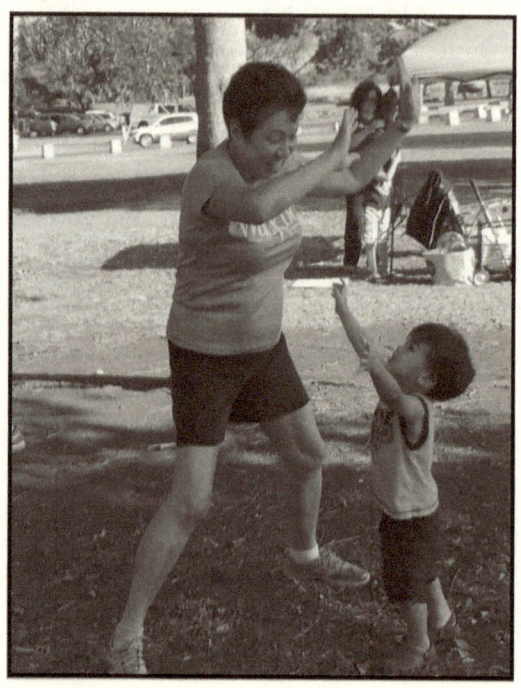

T hank goodness it is Friday, everyone. I don't know about you, but I am looking forward to the weekend. I want to share with you a significant concern that has recently come to my attention.

Understandably, many parents have feared bringing their children into doctors' offices and possibly exposing them to illnesses. However, by cancelling their child's well-child visits and vaccines, public health experts say this is starting to sow the seeds of another health crisis. As immunization rates drop, we are now putting millions of children and adults at risk for measles, whooping cough, and other deadly, but preventable, diseases. This is the last thing we need – collateral damage from this COVID-19 pandemic.

Many pediatric practices, like my own, have been adjusting office procedures to make it as safe as possible for patients to come in. Some of the changes include screening every call that comes in, scheduling well-child visits in the morning and sick visits in the afternoon, reserving one or two rooms solely for sick visits and maintaining the strictest sanitization of every room after each office visit.

Additionally, many families are under a great deal of stress with everyone at home, and this could be a recipe for disaster. We need to keep a close eye on the children and help all families navigate this stressful period.

Please remember to keep your child's annual or regularly scheduled visit appointment. Most pediatricians are still open and prepared to serve you and your family. Please share this vital information with others because delaying vaccinations indefinitely starts to put our entire community at greater risk for vaccine-preventable diseases.

I hope all of you have a fantastic weekend and try to make some "great mems" with your family.

> *"The Lord bless you and keep you; the Lord make his face to shine upon you and be gracious to you; the Lord turn his face toward you and give you peace."*
>
> —NUMBERS 6:24–26 NIV

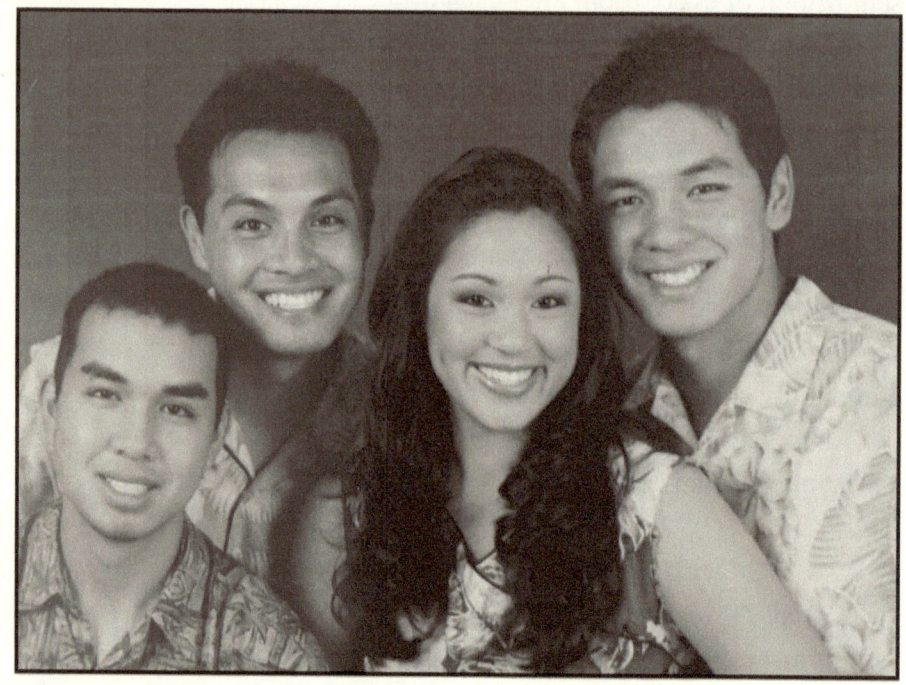

Happy Saturday, dear readers!

I am still listening to the John Maxwell audio book CD, entitled "The 360 Degree Leader," that I mentioned. He is such an uplifting and inspirational speaker, and I hope you'll check out some of his many books or podcasts. In this CD, he discusses the importance of knowing yourself and the unique gifts that only you possess. He encourages us to develop our talents or "sweet spot" and live the mission for which we were created, helping others with our God-given abilities.

Yesterday, I sat down to write about my unique talent and mission. My mission in life is to give families hope, encouragement, and simple tools to achieve their best health. I realize that change is never easy, but doing it together, as a family, makes it so much more attainable. In today's world, there is a wealth of conflicting information on how to achieve good health. Social media is constantly bombarding us with ads for expensive miracle diets or programs that ultimately fail to deliver. The thought I want each of you to ponder.

About today, it is never too late to get healthier. There's a saying that "health is your greatest wealth," and it's something that money cannot buy. So, consider taking that first step toward better health, regardless of your current stage in life. Let me give you an example of what this looks like. If your family enjoys having a sugar-sweetened beverage daily, consider setting a goal to decrease it to every other day for a week. Instead, replace this with milk or water, and if that works well, consider advancing it to one sweetened beverage every other day. Studies now show that sugar-sweetened beverages are the number one cause of obesity for our children. Not only will this simple goal benefit them, but the adults will also benefit greatly.

God has many plans for us, and we must take care of ourselves to live the fulfilled life God intended for us.

> *"So, whether you eat or drink, or whatever you do, do all for the glory of God."*
>
> —1 CORINTHIANS 10:31 NIV

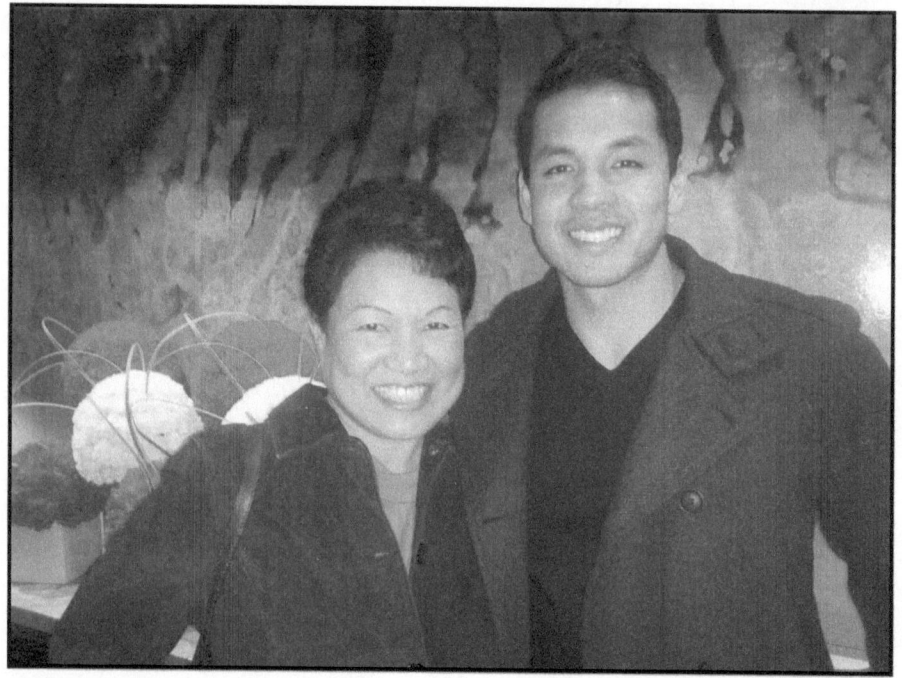

think what I miss most during this COVID-19 social distancing is the freedom to visit my children or grandchildren. Skyping them is just not the same. I wanted to share a little bit about my second son, Christopher Allen Wee. We were blessed with four children, and each had a unique personality.

Chris was born on November 4, just two years and two days after his older brother's birthday, November 2. For the first eight years of their lives, we were able to have combined birthday parties until they started to wise up to this situation. Chris was a great child because he could frequently entertain himself. He would sit for hours playing with Legos or taking a toy apart and then putting it back together. He was intelligent and quick-witted, but also impulsive, and struggled to control his comments and actions. My husband and I received frequent calls from the school on his behalf, and this soon became exhausting for us after a while.

No one said raising children was an easy task, and yes, there were times when I wanted to scream and pull my hair out. However, there were also many moments of reassurance from family, friends, and even teachers, who told me that he would be fine. On a few occasions, people would even come up and tell me that Chris was considered their favorite of all the Wee children. So, like his parents, we stayed on the course and hoped for the best. In his later high school years, Chris began to excel after identifying his strengths, and after a few more years growing up.

What I am most proud of in Chris is his desire to be independent and explore his life's calling. After graduating from the University of Hawaii with a business degree, he realized business was not for him after working at a desk job in this field. He announced to us one day that he was leaving for LA to attend EMT school. He supported himself as a waiter while attending school and living on his own, which helped him excel in "adulting." He finally returned to Hawaii and found love with his former high school classmate Samantha Robertson. They recently married, and to my surprise, Chris has shown all of us what a loving husband and father he is. As his dad would often say, "He has truly blossomed into a fine young man." Chris and Sam are expecting their second child in two months, and I couldn't be happier for them.

To all parents with young children out there, it seems like they will never grow up, but time does fly by quickly, and before you know it, they are on their own. Be patient and kind to them and show them how much you love them. Never lose hope. Tell them often how special they are to you. Most important of all, be present with them and make great memories together, for they are only on loan to us for a short time.

"Children are a heritage from the Lord, offspring a reward from him. Like arrows in the hands of a warrior are children born in one's youth. Blessed is the man whose quiver is full of them. They will not be put to shame when they contend with their opponents in court."

—PSALMS 127:3–5 NIV

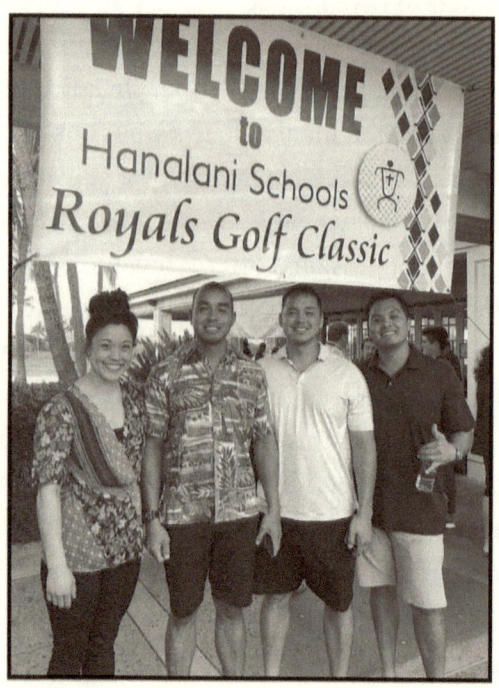

This pandemic has made me miss seeing my children and grandchildren in person. These lockdowns have made it even more critical to FaceTime or call them regularly to stay in touch. I recently touched base with my third son, Bradley Jonathan Wee, and it was so lovely to hear his voice. Stephen and I had always talked about having three or four children in our family. After my second son was born in 1986, I experienced a miscarriage, and it hit me very hard. I later realized that this is not that uncommon, but no one ever talks about it. I felt many emotions at that time, like sadness, guilt, confusion, and whether I might even be able to have more children.

You can imagine our emotions when we found out that I was expecting again. We were elated, yet cautious, but everything went well, and on July 15, 1987, Brad was born. We were overjoyed to welcome our third son into the family.

Brad was so adorable, and no one could resist pinching those chubby cheeks. He was easy-going, rarely cried, and generally very well behaved. However, if you crossed the line, he would let you and everyone else know it by striking back. Brad was "stealth," which meant that you would frequently forget he was around, then he would suddenly seize an opportunity and jump in from nowhere. His teachers would give us the same report each year. He never raised his hand in class, but when called upon, he always had the correct answer.

Brad was probably the most athletically skilled of the three Wee boys. He developed a keen interest in skateboarding at a young age and practiced whenever possible. He was never interested in traditional school sports. He also excelled in Xbox games, even though we never had one at home. However, he knew how to make friends and frequently visited our neighbors' houses.

One day, out of nowhere, he announced to me that he was joining the Hawaii Air National Guard and leaving for Officer Training School in Alabama. How could this neophyte hop into the military and become an officer? To my amazement, he graduated as a second lieutenant and then went to Florida for intense training as an air battle manager at Tyndall Air Force Base. Once again, he graduated to become an elite member of this group.

Brad continues to make me so proud. He is now a captain working full-time in the Hawaii Air National Guard. He loves his job and his country and is always striving to be the best in his career. He has come a long way from being my skateboarder, videogame player, and the son who once asked me, "What's wrong with a C in school?" Brad has already volunteered for deployment and eagerly accepts any opportunities, both nationally and abroad, to gain more experience. My third son has come a long way, and I know God has great plans for him.

"Children, obey your parents in the Lord, for this is right. 'Honor your father and mother' which is the first commandment with a promise – so that it may go well with you, and that you may enjoy long life on the earth."

—EPHESIANS 6:1–3 NIV

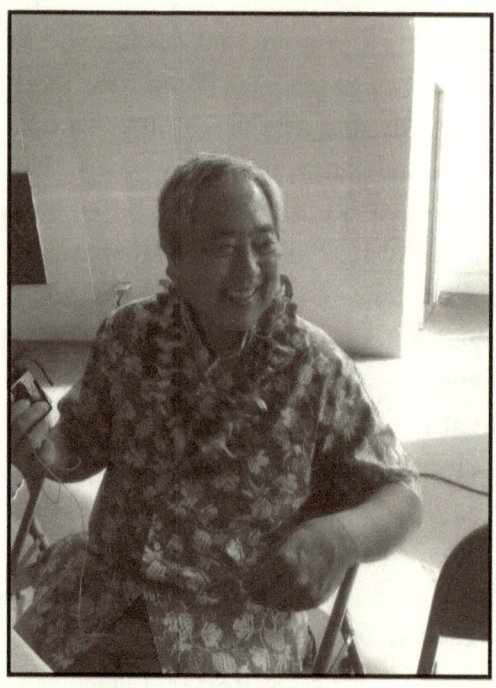

Dear readers, I have been weaving my faith into my blogs, and during this pandemic, my faith in God has become even stronger. It seems to me that when we have complex challenges, our faith in God becomes tested, and we either move further away or lean into and trust Him more. I have chosen to trust in God more, and today I wanted to share with you a very important person who has recently given me much inspiration and hope. His name is Pastor Jerry Higashi.

I attended Maryknoll school from an early age, listened to the nuns, learned my catechism, and even got confirmed. In college at UH Manoa, I got distracted with my intense pre-med and medical school studies, but kept the faith. I even ventured to attend Protestant services with "Campus Ministries."

Once married, Stephen, a baptized Protestant, agreed to have our entire family attend weekly Mass and catechism class. The children attended a Protestant non-denominational school nearby, so occasionally, things could be a little confusing to a young child. Nevertheless, life was good, and no matter which denomination you believe in, I always knew God had our backs.

My faith wavered significantly after the sudden and unexpected death of my husband at the age of fifty-five in 2010. I could not comprehend how a loving God could do this to such a good person. It just did not make sense. I stopped going to Church for months, not even believing there could be a loving God, until one night, I got down on my knees and pleaded with Him to show me a sign of what to do next. He provided me with my answer within five days, assigned me an experienced office manager, and together, we were able to revive my medical practice from the ashes. God then sent me Martin, who later became my husband. Through his encouragement, I soon began attending church once again, as well as an extraordinary small group meeting with him every week.

Just as my newly built office was up and running smoothly, I had to pause to undergo my third knee arthroscopy. As the only physician working at the office, I returned to work a few days after surgery and soon found myself back in the hospital, not only with a septic knee but also with bacteria in my blood. This was when I panicked and knew that people die of blood sepsis.

At this point, Pastor Jerry Higashi, only a distant acquaintance at that time, pulled up a chair and sat down by my side. During his visit, he listened intently as I just rambled on. To my surprise, I began to verbalize my fear of dying, my unfulfilled dreams, and my hope of starting a non-profit organization, Walk with a Doc – Oahu, and restarting my movement to make families healthier. Heck, I barely knew this guy, but this hospital visit left an impact on me I'll never forget.

I made a full recovery after being at home for two months on IV antibiotics. Doctors told me I was extremely "lucky," but I believe God had a hand in this and was not done with me yet.

I slowly got to know Pastor Jerry through acquaintances and even visited his small church a few times. He always seemed to be there for me during some of the most deeply challenging times. His calm manner and expert listening skills have encouraged and uplifted me to keep pressing forward. He has helped me to search Scripture and have an even more meaningful relationship with God. Martin and I now attend his church regularly every Sunday.

Through all my challenges, my faith in God has been strengthened with each trial, including this coronavirus pandemic. I now view challenges as opportunities and no longer ask why, but rather how I can use them to learn more about myself and help others in the process. Today, during my time of pause, I want to express my gratitude to Pastor Jerry for being by my side through it all.

> *"As iron sharpens iron, so one person sharpens another. He who tends a fig tree will eat its fruit, and he who looks after His master will be honored. As water reflects a face, so a man's heart reflects the man."*
>
> —PROVERBS 27:17–19 NIV

ENTRY: 04/30/20

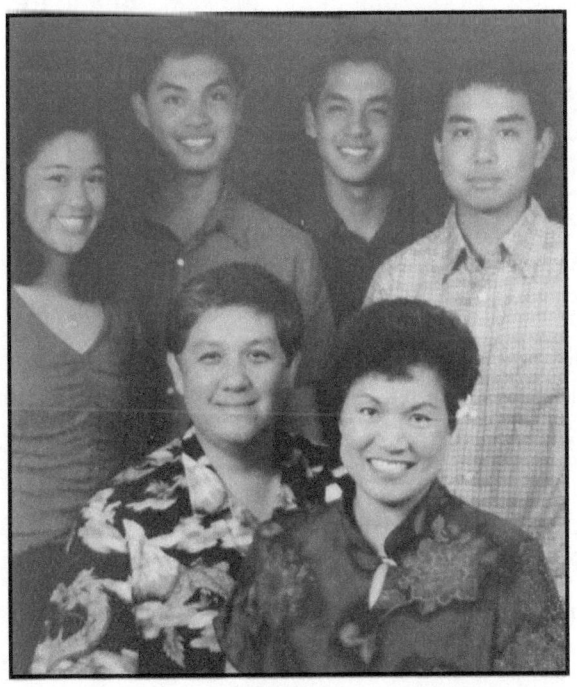

had a team meeting this morning with my office staff. During this pandemic, numerous moving parts necessitate daily adjustments. They certainly did not teach me this in medical school, but my learning curve has been very steep recently. These weekly meetings have been crucial in reviewing our daily workflows, ensuring everyone is consistent with the new routine of sanitizing the office after each patient. These meetings have also served as an excellent outlet and forum for communicating concerns and fears. To my surprise, my staff are very concerned about getting COVID-19, and they appreciate the extra steps I am taking to keep everyone safe. My primary goal is to provide the best care for our patients and families, while also ensuring the safety and well-being of my entire staff, including myself.

With this coronavirus pandemic always on our minds, I wanted to share with you an important lesson I've learned from my grief journey and how I am applying this to what we are all experiencing right now.

When my husband passed, the main question that kept repeating in my head was How was I going to live the next thirty to forty years without him? Could I ever be happy again? Could I ever travel the world as we had planned? At the time, I could only see the distant future through glasses tinted with despair and hopelessness.

To help me answer some of these probing questions, I must share with you, dear readers, that I found my strength to move forward and find out through a monthly grief support group. I wasn't even sure what this was or if I needed it, but a friend suggested it might help, so I was open to trying it once.

As I sat in my first meeting, I realized for the first time that I was not the only one experiencing a significant loss, and I finally felt that I wasn't going crazy. I now found myself among people who understood, accepted, and validated my feelings. They surrounded me with love and understanding. These grief support meetings gave me so much comfort that I continued attending these monthly meetings for the past ten years.

As new people joined the group and shared their losses, I continued to experience great healing just by sharing my story and coming alongside them. I have learned so much in these past ten years about myself as well as learning that by helping others, you help yourself even more. This grief journey I am on will always be a part of me. There is still great sorrow in knowing that Stephen is no longer here, but also enormous gratitude for the many years we spent together. My husband shaped me into the person that I am today, and I will forever be grateful. As I move forward in life, I feel him beside me and cheering me on. I know he would have wanted me to be happy and find my way in this second phase of my life.

In stressful times like these, I genuinely believe that we need to be in the here and now more than ever. Things like my morning cup of coffee, daily walks outdoors, a surprise Skype visit with my grandchildren – these are the moments that I find wonderful and need to appreciate for all their goodness fully. Groucho Marx is quoted as saying, "Yesterday is dead, tomorrow hasn't arrived yet. I have just one day, today, and I'm going to be happy in it."

So, dear readers, use this precious time to be present in the moment and reconnect with your family. We cannot let the wonderful moments slip away from us, even during this pandemic.

"Write it on your heart that every day is the best day in the year."

—RALPH WALDO EMERSON

"There is a time for everything, and a season for every activity under heaven: a time to be born and a time to die, a time to plant and a time to uproot, a time to kill and a time to heal, a time to tear down and a time to build, a time to weep and a time to laugh, a time to mourn and a time to dance, a time to scatter stones and a time to gather them, a time to embrace and a time to refrain, a time to search and a time to give up, a time to keep and a time to throw away, a time to tear and a time to mend, a time to be silent and a time to speak, a time to love and a time to hate, a time for war and a time for peace."

—ECCLESIASTES 3:1–8 NIV

3

MAY

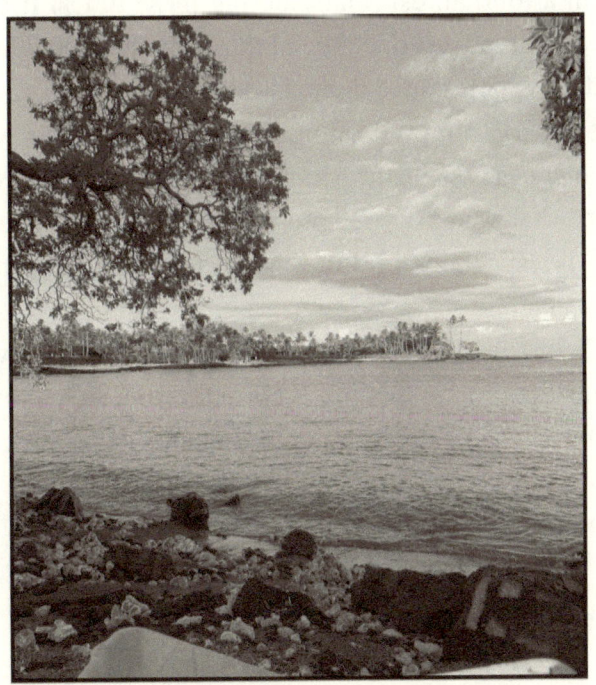

Today is May 1, and "May Day is Lei Day" in Hawaii. Traditionally, our schools, community, and other groups would have gatherings and Spring Programs with an abundance of fresh leis and flowers. However, with our current COVID-19 pandemic, we can only post pictures of our flower leis on social media or perhaps display them on our front doors. Nevertheless, I feel grateful to live in one of the most beautiful places on earth.

Today, as I look back on this past month, I have been pleasantly surprised that I have been consistent with my blogs and never seem to run out of things to share with you, my dear readers.

I have decided to continue this writing journey and hope you find some information, humor, and inspiration on these various topics. I am deeply humbled and encouraged by the touching comments many of you have shared with me about what these blogs have meant to you.

Therefore, my homework to all of you is to think about writing your daily blogs in a journal, especially during these times. It doesn't have to be lengthy, perhaps just one crucial thing that happened to you today. Several medical articles have demonstrated that journaling is beneficial for one's health. By simply writing down your thoughts and feelings, you can manage stress better, improve your immune system, keep your memory sharp, boost your mood, and strengthen your emotional health. This is especially true during these challenging times of the COVID-19 pandemic.

So, don't just sit there… start writing today! Don't worry about grammar, punctuation, or spelling. This is for you, so let your pen flow. I am sure you will soon start to reap the benefits of keeping a journal.

> *"He who was seated on the throne said, 'I am making everything new.' Then he said, 'Write this down, for these words are trustworthy and true."*
>
> —REVELATION 21:5 NIV

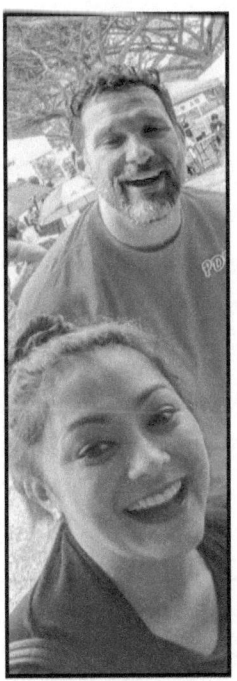

During the COVID-19 pandemic, I discovered the value of new technology. For the first time last night, I joined a most heart-warming "Instagram Live" Tenth Anniversary Celebration of the Pas de Deux Dance Studio. Wendy and Jeremy Gilbert started this dance studio in Waipahu ten years ago but let me tell you the rest of the story.

In 1993, when my daughter, Malia, was three and a half, Stephen and I saw a handwritten road sign announcing that dance classes were starting up at a nearby school. We decided to enroll her, as we both worked every Saturday morning. On the first day of class, Malia wore her favorite black dress and shoes. She took a leap and landed on her bottom, but to her credit, she dusted herself off and returned to the line. This marked the beginning of her lifelong love affair with dance, and she has continued dancing ever since. Her teacher was an entrepreneurial sixteen-year-old, Wendy Calio. She and her mom, Teresa Osthoff, were already making a positive difference in children's lives through the Sabrina Starr Dance Studio.

Since there were so many classes, practices, parades, and performances, Stephen and I relied heavily on the other families to help us with car rides. Our families were united by the common bond of our daughters dancing, and as a result, formed priceless, lifelong friendships in the process.

The studio's budget was minimal, and it was a labor of love. Sabrina Starr Dance Studio has moved five times. The only places we could afford were always in dire need of cleaning and renovating. I recall many nights when Stephen and I went to the studio from 9 PM to midnight to work. We even got to know the night guards. Stephen would do repairs, paint, make set decorations, and do whatever Wendy asked for.

Together, through blood, sweat, and tears, the entire dance family rolled up their sleeves and transformed dilapidated spaces that no one wanted to rent into a paradise for dancers. For several years, Wendy went away to pursue other dreams, but Stephen and I, by then, unofficially "adopted" her and continued to assist her.

In 2009, we met up again with Wendy and Jeremy in Beverly Hills, California, and listened intently as she shared her dreams of returning home to open a new dance studio. Stephen immediately jumped on the bandwagon and began encouraging and brainstorming with them. And the rest, as they say, is history. This was the birth of Pas de Deux Studio in 2010.

One moment that stood out for me about the studio occurred on Friday, June 11, 2010, which began like any other ordinary day. Stephen and I saw patients in the office that morning, then we had planned to spend the afternoon at the dance studio to place another dance floor. Stephen never made it there and passed away that afternoon. Word spread quickly, and soon other dance dads were there at the studio to complete the job.

Last night, I sat there listening to the many students, parents, and teachers talk about their favorite memories and moments of Pas de Deux over the past decade, and I couldn't help but think of the positive impact Wendy and Jeremy have had on the youth of Hawaii. They continue a legacy of shaping our young generation into solid, young adults who learn great values such as hard work, grit, compassion, and empathy. I feel so honored to have been a small part of this, and I know Stephen is so proud of all their efforts.

We love you, Wendy and Jeremy, and pray that God will continue to bless you and your business always.

> *"He took a little child whom he placed among them. Taking the child in his arms, he said to them, 'Whoever welcomes one of these little children in my name welcomes me; and whoever welcomes me does not welcome me but the one who sent me.'"*

—MARK 9:36–37

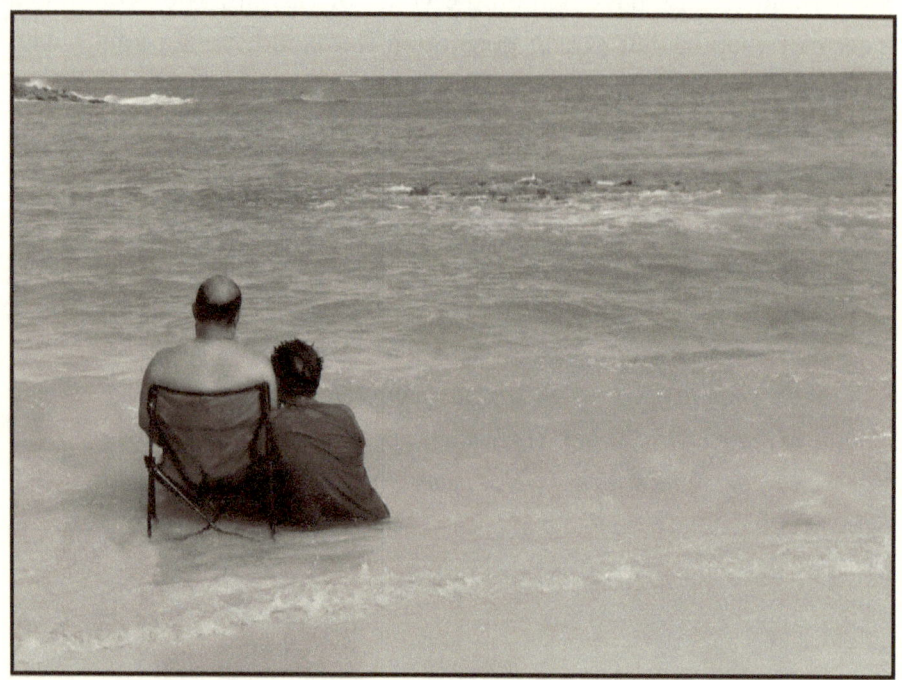

T oday, after our virtual church service, we decided to go for a swim in the ocean. It was such a beautiful, sunny day, and I had to break the monotony of the week. Being there was such an exhilarating experience that I wanted to share it with you. For a moment, I forgot all about the coronavirus pandemic.

My visit to the ocean today felt like a symbolic cleansing of my mind and body. This was my first visit to the sea in months. I cannot even remember the last time I swam at any beach this year. It felt so good to allow my entire body to relax in the water, feel the warmth of the sun on my face, and the waves gently rocking me back and forth in weightlessness. I felt like a baby being caressed in her mother's loving arms.

The sound of the repetitive, whooshing ocean waves seemed to keep telling me, "Don't worry, don't worry, everything is going to be okay." I could feel calmness overcome me and whatever anxieties I had, seemed to melt away during those moments in the water. I was mindful of my breathing, the waves coming one after another, the sand and rocks beneath my feet, the laughter of children on the beach, and my husband by my side.

As we drove home, I felt both exhausted and energized simultaneously. We spent over an hour in the water, as well as walking along the sandy beaches. After lunch and drinking a lot of water, we both had a great Sunday afternoon nap. I'm so ready for the week to start tomorrow, and I plan to make this a weekly ritual from now on. I forgot how healing a swim in the ocean can be.

I know there are many of you, my dear readers, feeling anxious or depressed from months of social isolation due to the COVID-19 pandemic, but my recommendation to you is to spend just an hour at the beach or simply outdoors. This will be an hour well spent, and I promise you won't regret it.

"This is what the Lord says, he who appoints the sun to shine by night, who stirs up the sea so that the waves roar – the Lord Almighty is his name."

—JEREMIAH 31:35 NIV

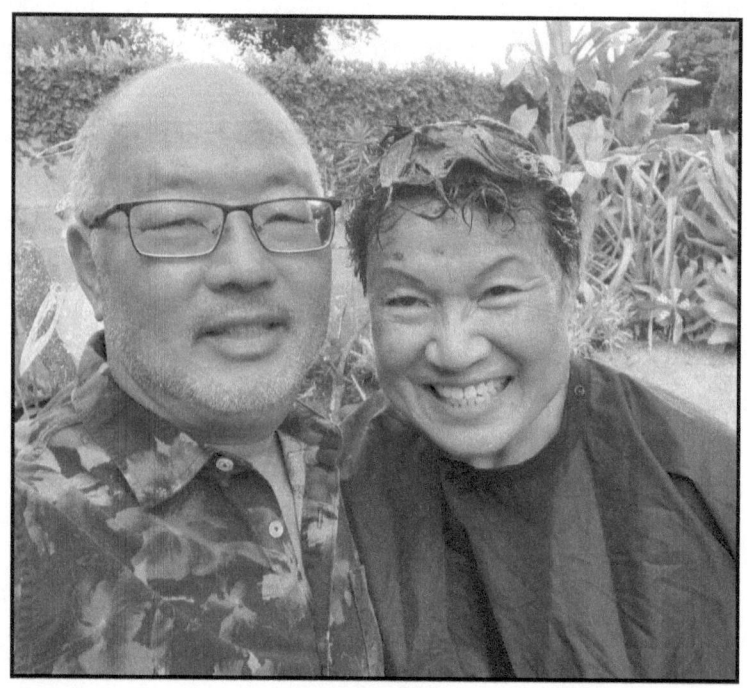

When I first heard about the coronavirus outbreak in China, I never thought it would ever affect me here in Hawaii. However, the truth is that quarantine and social distancing became a reality for all of us worldwide, turning our lives upside down.

I wanted to share with you some surprising things I have learned about myself during this period.

The first thing I learned is that it's okay to have some downtime alone. I don't always need every minute scheduled for a task. I have been enjoying a slower pace at home and in the office. It has been nice to take the time to read books I have always meant to read, sleep in if I feel like it, and listen to podcasts of my choosing.

I have learned that I enjoy being outdoors, whether it is at the beach, on my daily evening walks, or just sitting in my backyard. The weeds are gone, the bushes are trimmed, the plants have been repotted, and the tomatoes have been harvested. I appreciate the calm trade winds, the beautiful flowers, the birds that visit daily, and the breathtaking sunsets that have recently been a delight.

I have also realized that I don't need too many material things. I have been on a mission to declutter my belongings, including clothes, books, and other items that I no longer need or that no longer bring me joy. I have them all boxed up and ready to donate as soon as this pandemic eases up. It has been liberating and refreshing to get rid of excess and know that I have enough and am grateful for what I do have.

With all the new opportunities to be at home, I have found myself becoming more creative. I have been enjoying my time journaling and writing down my thoughts and feelings in a free-flowing manner. It has been a new experience for me to create a new blog daily and share from my heart. I have also become creative with my cooking, trying new recipes, making my greeting cards, and even updating my home computer, which had been neglected. I feel like I am learning to make the most of what I already have. Before the pandemic, I would have gone to the store.

I've learned many things about myself, and it's been a lot of fun exploring them. I have had time to appreciate how blessed I am. I never want to take for granted my family, staff, friends, good health, and so much more. God is good, all the time!

Speaking of blessings, I am so blessed to have a husband who is always willing to help me with just about any requests I have. Yesterday, I asked in the sweetest voice if he could help me buzz trim and then dye my hair. He immediately rolled up his sleeves and even read the instructions on the dye box. (He never reads directions, but I think he didn't want to make a mistake.)

I'm happy to report that he did a fantastic job, and I saved a significant amount of money. The next task for him will be a pedicure and painting my nails. I'll let you know how that goes. I think he may have found his second calling as a stylist! Ladies, he's not taking appointments yet.

"Love is patient, love is kind. It does not envy, it does not boast, it is not proud. It does not dishonor others, it is not self-seeking, it is not easily angered, it keeps no record of wrongs."

—1 CORINTHIANS 13:4–5 NIV

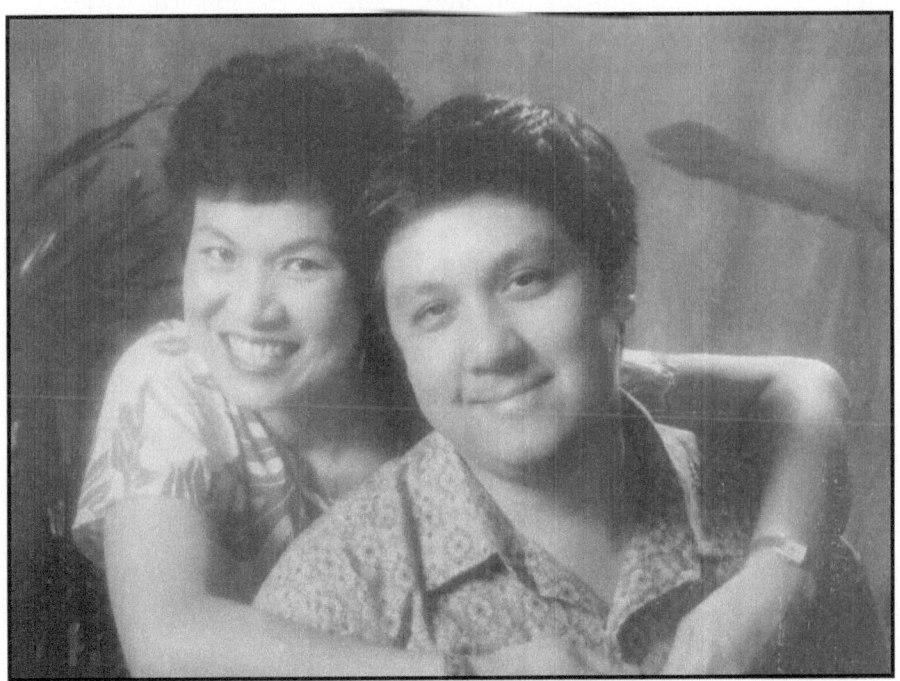

D espite the ongoing pandemic, I am still able to continue seeing our patients for their well-child visits in the office and keep them up to date on their vaccines. For children with fevers and other symptoms, we are conducting these visits via telehealth. Some physician offices have closed their doors completely and are only offering telehealth visits.

I want to share an encounter I had yesterday with a dear friend of many years. He was my husband's patient, and it was lovely to hear him recall how Stephen and I had touched his family. He went on to say that as he sat in my waiting room, he told his son about my husband and the journey I have been on since his death. He said he wanted him to know how my life story had unfolded and how proud he was of me.

Sometimes, simply sharing a story or a few words about how someone has touched your life can be an uplifting and beautiful gift to someone who has lost a loved one. It means that their life meant something, and they are still remembered. I am always thankful whenever I am stopped by one of Stephen's former patients, many of whom are strangers to me, who share from their heart what his care as a physician meant to them.

Discussing the death of a loved one is an uncomfortable topic for many. Perhaps it reminds them of their mortality, or that feeling of intense grief and pain makes it painful for them to listen.

For me, after being in group grief support, I have learned that no matter how hard it is to talk about our loss, it is not only beneficial but healing as well. By confronting my anger, loss, and sadness, I have dealt with all these emotions better. It is cathartic to release these emotions in words and tears, knowing that you are not alone in feeling this way. I knew I wanted to move forward and not stay stuck in this very dark valley. I wanted something positive to come out of this personal tragedy. I genuinely believe that if I had suppressed it all, it would only fester and cause more physical damage, emotionally and mentally, later down the road.

The takeaway from this, then, is to take a bold step and reach out to someone who is mourning a loss and being by their side. Write or call them and see if it's okay to talk with them about their departed loved one. I know they would appreciate hearing stories about their loved ones and the impact they had on them.

I am deeply grateful to the many people around me who have shared their cherished memories of the beloved Dr. Stephen Wee, as well as to those who have listened to me talk about the incredible legacy of love that Stephen left behind. By walking directly out of this deep valley, with God by my side, I feel that I have emerged on the other end a stronger and better person. In grief support, we call ourselves "wounded warriors" because, despite the tragedy of losing a loved one, we learn a great deal from this and then pay it forward by helping others in their journey through grief.

"So, with you: Now is your time of grief, but I will see you again, and you will rejoice, and no one will take away your joy. On that day, you will no longer ask me anything. Very truly I tell you, my Father will give you whatever you ask in my name."

—JOHN 16:22–23 NIV

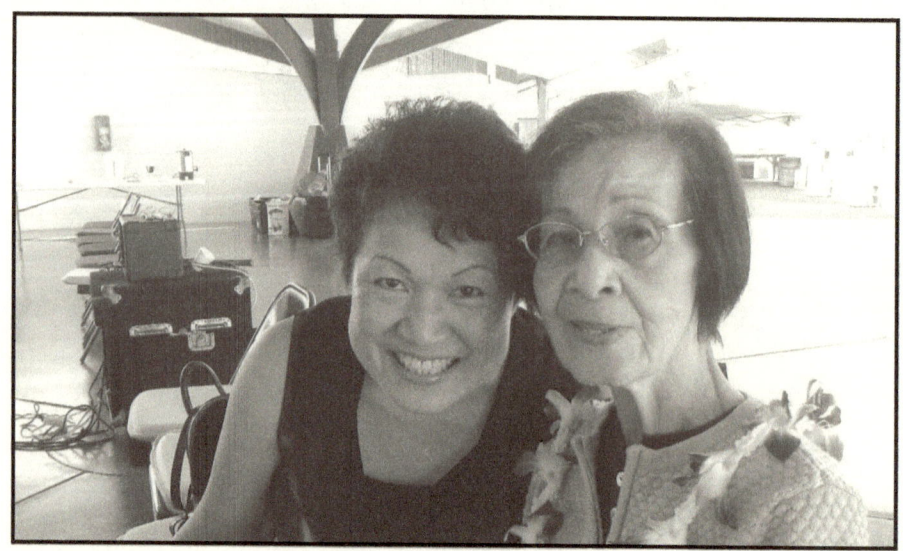

As we approach Mother's Day this coming Sunday, I've had a lot of time to think about the many challenges expectant mothers, new mothers, and all mothers are facing during this pandemic. As mothers, we always want what is best for our children, but in these uncertain times, we must all make decisions that we believe are in their best interest, based on the information available to us.

As I think about Mother's Day, I can't help but recollect memories of my mother, who I felt also did the best she could.

Mom was born in the mid-1920s, during the Great Depression years. I recall hearing stories about how my maternal grandparents would make large pots of soup and feed neighbors who didn't have enough to eat. I certainly admire how kind and generous they were. My maternal grandparents barely had an elementary school education. Despite this, the importance of education was always stressed in my parents' families, and it continued into our generation.

My mother excelled in high school and eventually earned her master's degree in social work from Boston University. There, she met and married my dad, who was also from Hawaii, and graduated from MIT with a master's degree in Structural Engineering. They returned home. After my mom had four children, she decided to stop working outside the home and became a full-time, stay-at-home mom. In addition, she also cared for my maternal grandparents, who also lived with us.

As a young girl, I always craved her attention, but I soon learned that she rarely gave out praise. I now understand that she was always proud of me, as I always heard stories from her friends about me. It was okay, though, because my dad would always lavish me with those positive and encouraging words.

Before my mom passed away in 2013, I thanked her often for the sacrifices she made and how appreciative I was of her. Through Martin's urging, she eventually agreed to come to our church regularly, and four months before her death, she accepted Jesus into her heart and was baptized.

As I look back, there were many things she and my dad could have done better, but as a parent myself, I know that none of us are perfect. We keep moving forward, doing our best and loving our children unconditionally.

So, to all the mothers and the mothers-to-be out there, motherhood is probably the most challenging job you will ever have, but it will also be the most rewarding. I wish each of you God's protection, guiding hand, and love be upon you and your family always. Happy Mother's Day, 2020!

"Listen to your father, who gave you life, and do not despise your mother when she is old. Buy the truth and do not sell it; get wisdom, discipline, and understanding. The father of a righteous man has great joy; he who has a wise son delights in him. May your father and mother be glad; may she who gave birth rejoice!"

—PROVERBS 23:22–25 NIV

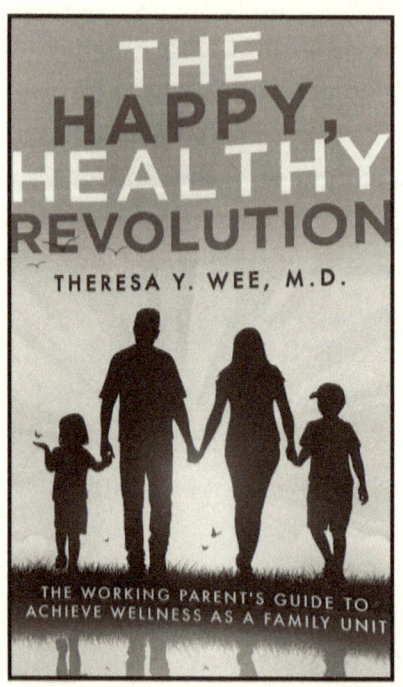

I recently completed my first book, entitled *The Happy, Healthy Revolution: A Working Parents' Guide to Achieve Wellness as a Family*. During the COVID-19 pandemic, I realized that many parents are currently at home, and this may be the perfect time to consider drawing ideas from my book to help you and your family achieve better health.

I am also committed to recording my audiobook, rather than having someone else read it. As the author, I knew this manuscript better than anyone else and was confident that I could do the best job. I finally received the call several weeks ago, informing me that it was now time to start recording my audiobook.

I received a large, professional microphone in the mail and was required to record in my bedroom, where the sound would be dampened, which would produce the best sound quality. After several days of trial and error in setting it up, I was finally able to start recording, thanks to the help of my patient husband.

I have now completed recording nearly half of my book, and this task is not as easy as it looks. After reading the entire book, I believe that much of the information contained therein can greatly benefit many families currently in lockdown. My book will take you and your family step by step on how to make small but meaningful changes that can eventually add up to significant results, learn the secret to maintaining healthy changes for a lifetime, and understand ways to set individual and family goals that lead to more family connectedness as well as better physical and emotional well-being.

The most important aspect of my approach is that the entire family must be fully committed and ready to make changes together. This is the key to success, with everyone in the house working toward a common goal and keeping one another accountable. As I keep telling my families, teamwork is so much better, and together, everyone can achieve so much more.

Please share this information with a family member, loved one, or friend who may need assistance in this area.

> *"Husbands, in the same way be considerate as you live with your wives and treat them with respect as the weaker partner and as heirs with you of the gracious gift of life, so that nothing will hinder your prayers. Finally, all of you live in harmony with one another; be sympathetic, love one another as brothers, be compassionate, and humble. Do not repay evil with evil or insult with insult, [but] with blessing, because to this you were called so that you may inherit a blessing."*
>
> —1 PETER 3:7–9 NIV

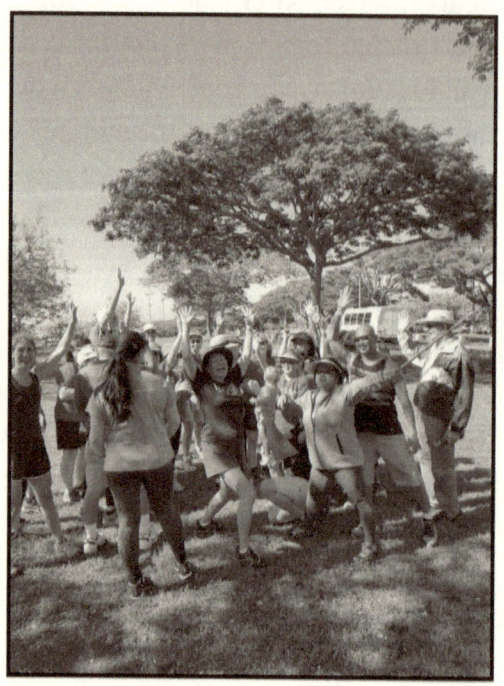

With more free time on hand, I've been able to reach out to dear friends from afar – from Molokai to the East Coast. It feels so good to spend time catching up with one another. Today, I wanted to share with you this TED Talk by Robert Waldinger, from 2015, which I viewed today, and I believe it has a lot of relevance to our current time. It reveals why it is so Important to take time and reach out, especially if someone is very isolated and lonely.

Mr. Waldinger is one of several generations of researchers who continue to work on the seventy-five-year-long "Harvard Study of Adult Development," which began in 1938. They gathered two groups of men: one group consisted of Harvard sophomores, and the other group comprised men from the impoverished Boston tenements. The goal of this study was to identify the factors that contribute to people's happiness and overall well-being throughout their lifetime. Today, sixty of the

124 men are still alive, and they continue to send out questionnaires every year, as well as conduct interviews with their wives, children, and grandchildren. Many of these men are now in their nineties. These are the three main lessons they have learned thus far:

- Social connections are crucial for maintaining your overall health. The more connected you are, the healthier you are, and the longer you are likely to live. They also found that loneliness kills, and the less happy you are, the earlier you will die.
- The quality of your relationship is of great importance. It is not the actual number of friends you have or whether you are in a committed relationship. What is much more important is that you are in a good and nourishing relationship. When they checked in on these men at age fifty, they found it was not their cholesterol level that indicated whether they would be healthy in later years, but rather how satisfied they were with their relationships that mattered.
- Good relationships protect not only our bodies, but also our brains. When we are in a secure, attached relationship in our eighties, our memories stay sharper. These relationships did not have to be smooth sailing all the time, but if each partner knew they could count on one another, that's what mattered.

The overwhelming conclusion of this ongoing study is that good close relationships are essential not only for our survival but also for the quality of our lives. I have a suggestion for this weekend: replace the screen time with people time. Do something special with a loved one or reach out to a family member or friend you haven't spoken to in a while.

Relationships are not always easy and can become complicated, but the bottom line is that investing in relationship building is worth it. Don't hold grudges; use this time during the pandemic and this Mother's Day weekend to let them go. Everyone will benefit and be blessed.

"A new commandment I give you: Love one another. As I have loved you, so must you love one another. By this everyone will know that you are my disciples if you love one another."

—JOHN 13:34–35 NIV

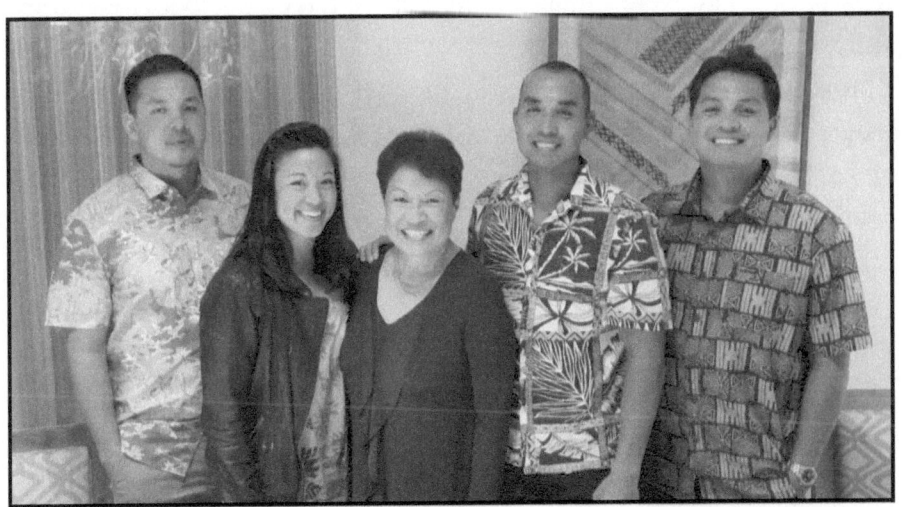

On this Mother's Day, I got to sleep in. My husband would have taken me out for brunch, but because of the pandemic, I decided to treat myself and place a takeout order. Today, I want to share with you, a "Special Letter" I wrote to my four children on this Mother's Day, as I am unable to celebrate it in person with them.

Dear David, Chris, Brad, and Stephanie Malia,

Today's blog is dedicated to the four of you. Thank you for all your early Mother's Day wishes. As I pause and reflect, I want you to know how blessed I feel to be your mother.

There were times when I thought all of you would never grow up, and then in an instant, you were off to college and on your own. I must admit that there were times when I felt like parenting was too much, but there were also many times when we created wonderful family memories. Even though Dad and I worked six days a week in our medical practices, we made a conscious effort to prioritize family time.

No one prepares you for parenthood, which I now see as my most important task in life. Dad and I tried to combine the best of our past experiences with our parents to come up with our parenting style. As I look back, there were things we both could have done better or differently, but no parent is perfect, and we tried to learn from our mistakes. I think we both always tried to do our best at the time. All four of you taught us what unconditional love means and how wonderful it felt to be part of a loving family.

Through the good times and bad, we made it, guys. I miss Dad so much, but he touched us with a special love. We will never forget him. He will always be in our hearts and have a special place there. I know for sure that he would have been so proud of each one of you.

Please continue to share your love with your family, friends, and anyone you encounter. I hope each of you continues to flourish and bring joy to those around you. I pray that God continues to bless you and keep you safe and healthy.

> *"So then, brothers and sisters stand firm and hold to the teachings we passed on to you, whether by word of mouth or by letter. May our Lord Jesus Christ himself and God our Father, who loved us and by his grace gave us eternal encouragement and good hope, encourage your hearts and strengthen you in every good deed and word."*
>
> —2 THESSALONIANS 2:15–17 NIV

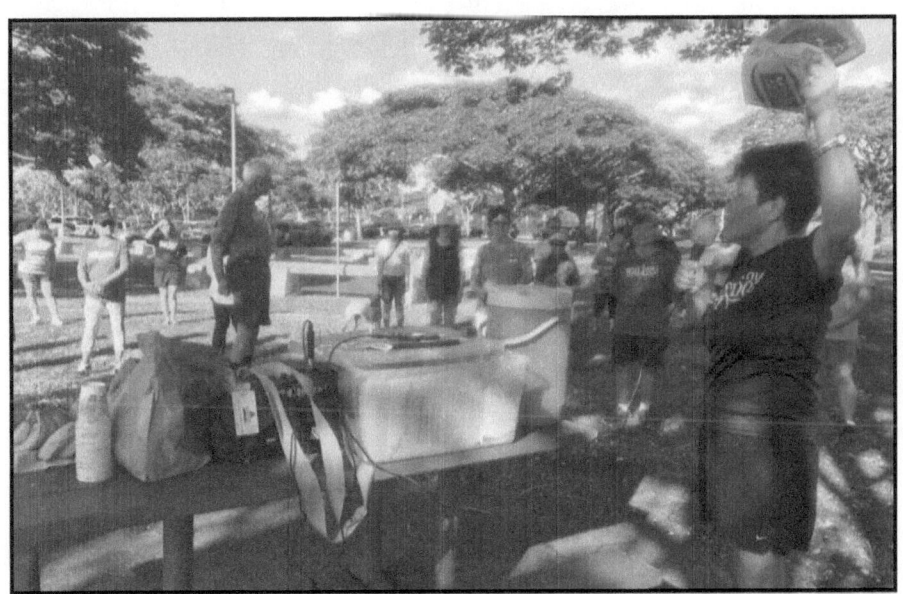

fter listening to this morning's COVID-19 briefings on television, I'm more confused than ever. As a physician, I consult with health experts, but they often disagree on the best course of action. In the final analysis, all this uncertainty is making our lives unpredictable and causing even more stress.

This resulting stress culminates in not only adverse physical responses, such as headaches or fatigue, but it also worsens pre-existing mental illness. It can trigger bouts of depression and anxiety. Additionally, stress has been shown to weaken our immune response, thus causing us to be more susceptible to illnesses, including the COVID-19 virus.

Therefore, each of us must find ways to manage our stress response, as this will help us stay healthy and improve the quality of our lives. Some things I have been trying to do daily are:

- Eating three balanced meals a day, with plenty of fruit and vegetables.

- Getting seven to eight hours of sleep a night and going to sleep at the same time consistently.
- Regular exercise, which includes walking 10,000 steps every evening with my husband and drinking water often.
- Ten minutes of quiet time in the morning and evening, praying, meditating, or simply reflecting.

As we move forward, we are entering a new era, a defining moment in our lives like no other. The coronavirus has brought our entire world to a literal standstill, affecting every aspect of our lives, including athletic events, entertainment, education, religion, media, elections, health, and much more.

This morning, my prayer was for the removal of all fear and doubts, and I asked God to replace them with hope and anticipation of something even greater to happen when this is all over. I hope to learn from this pandemic and personally emerge stronger, happier, and more compassionate.

I know that God loves us so much, and I am sure he has an ultimate plan for each of us in all of this. Let us all trust God and look to the future in expectation of even greater things to come.

> *"Peace, I leave you, my peace I give you. I do not give to you as the world gives you. Do not let your hearts be troubled and do not be afraid."*
>
> —JOHN 14:27 NIV

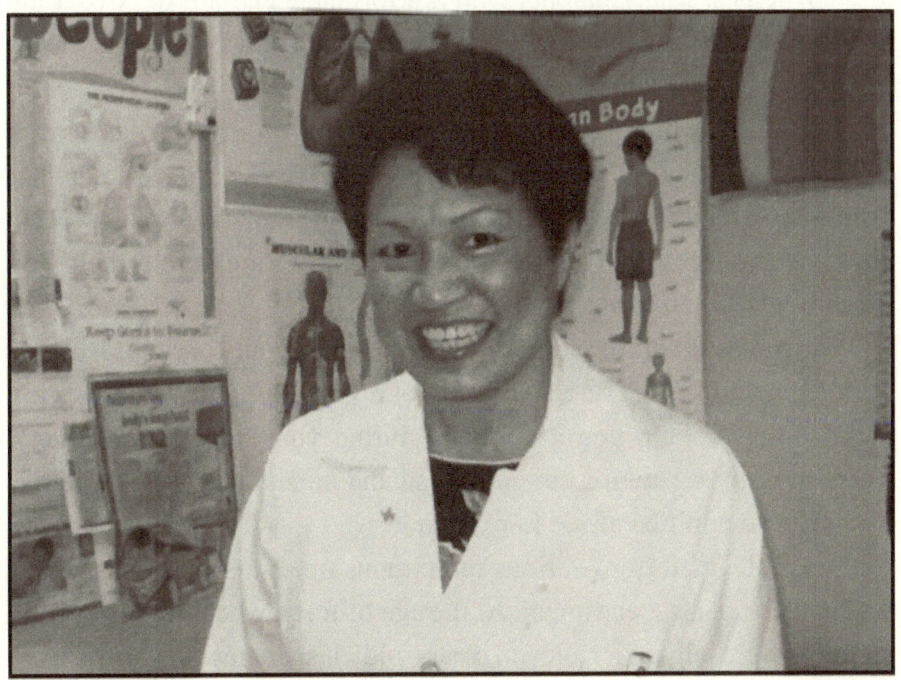

L ast night, I listened to a father's story about how he recently lost his twelve-year-old son to suicide during this COVID-19 quarantine time. There were a series of events that ultimately led to his tragic death. This dad truly believes that if his son were in school, with less free time and more engagement with his friends, this entire situation would have been avoided. This YouTube clip broke my heart and made me realize that this is only one example of the many collateral damages we'll start to hear about from this COVID-19 pandemic lockdown.

People of all ages are taking a hit and truly suffering emotionally. The significant toll this pandemic is taking on families is slowly coming to light. It was reported recently that the calls to suicide prevention centers and domestic hotlines have skyrocketed during April.

When I hear people saying that this COVID-19 lockdown is like an extended summer vacation, they are severely mistaken. Parents are losing their jobs, families are standing in food lines for the first time, children are not allowed to visit their friends, and everyone is confined to their homes. Many parents who are fortunate enough to have a job must also work from home and homeschool their children. By no means is this a vacation for anyone.

Tensions are high, and emotions are flying, so it won't take much to reach the breaking point. I encourage my readers to consult their primary care physician if they are experiencing similar symptoms. Most physicians' offices are open for business, and we are here to help you get through this challenging period.

When discussing the importance of reaching out for help, I like to use the analogy of a crutch. If you broke your leg, you would readily use a crutch to help you get around during your period of recovery. The same can be said for our emotional and mental well-being. Help is available, so don't be afraid to reach out.

What I learned from various tumultuous times in my life was that I was indeed not a superwoman. At the age of forty, when my four young children were all under eleven years old, I suddenly began to have difficulty falling asleep and staying asleep. I worked six days a week in my office and was on call 24/7. I not only had to care for my patients but also came home every day to my second full-time job: caring for my family and household. There was always something to do, such as grocery shopping, cooking, cleaning, laundry, and reviewing homework, among other tasks. I began to lose my appetite and, for over a year, struggled with just not feeling myself. One day, while reading my medical journal, I suddenly realized that I had all the symptoms of a major depressive episode. I immediately sought the help of a psychiatrist, and within weeks, I slowly emerged from this dark tunnel I had fallen into.

However, there is a silver lining to this dark experience that I would like to share with you. I finally understood that there was a limit to what one person can do, and sometimes it is necessary for our pride to step aside and accept help. After we all understood what I was going through, our family adjusted, and my husband and children had to contribute more to helping. We worked as a team, and it made our family stronger.

I also believe it made me a better pediatrician and opened my eyes to the needs of the families I care for daily.

This pandemic is indeed very difficult for many, but I want to encourage anyone experiencing deep hardships to at least talk to someone close or seek professional help. As parents and role models for our family, we need to show our children that these new challenges are opportunities for them to learn and grow. We can show our children that we are committed to showing up daily and working as a team to solve problems.

If we're accustomed to being the "helper," we may not feel comfortable in the role of the person who needs help. But sometimes our burdens are so significant that there is no way to deal with them alone. Thus, for this season, it's okay to be one of the "weak ones" who needs to be cared for. In another season, we will be the "strong ones" who care for others.

Life is all about taking turns caring for and, in turn, being cared for. That's just the way it is, and it's a natural part of being human. The journey of life is filled with many unpredictable twists and turns, as well as its share of ups and downs. As we walk along the road to recovery, let's watch for other travelers who may need help, just as we may need theirs.

> *"'Teacher, which is the greatest commandment in the Law?' Jesus replied: 'Love the Lord your God with all your heart and with all your soul and with all your mind. This is the first and greatest commandment. And the second is like it: Love your neighbor as yourself.'"*
>
> —MATTHEW 22:36–39 NIV

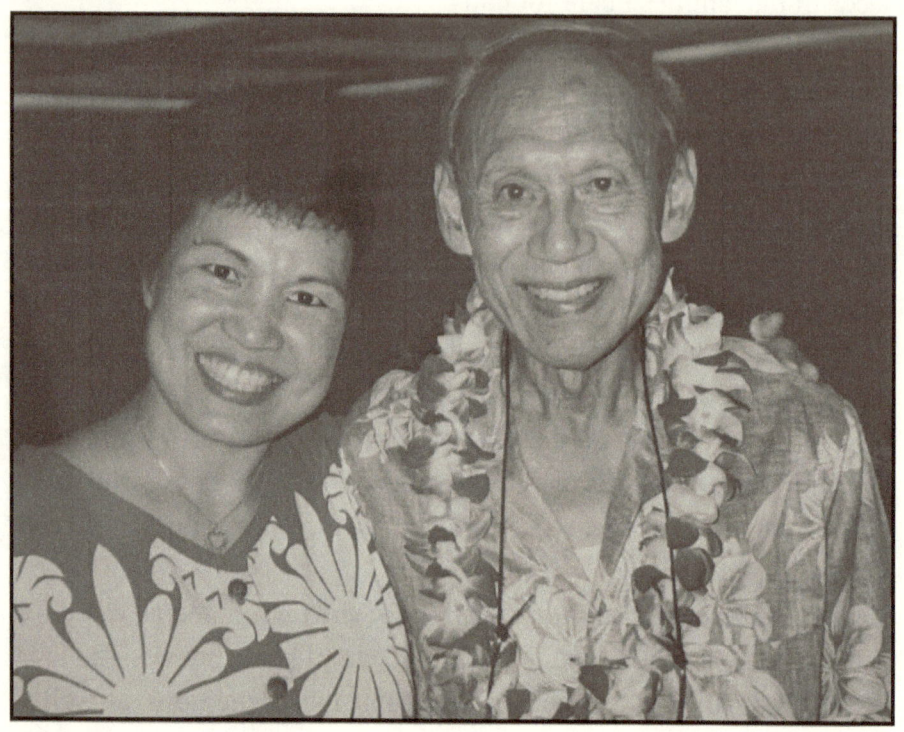

During this COVID-19 pandemic, most of us have been in lockdown with our families. Today, I sat down and began going through a box of old photos. It brought back so many memories that I wanted to share some insights about my own family from my childhood. I genuinely believe that the love of a family is life's greatest blessing.

I was the second of four children and sandwiched between two brothers. I always felt that I had to compete against them in sports or academics to get noticed. This was a self-imposed thought, but it motivated me to excel or at least try my best. My parents were extremely hard workers, and family time was limited. My dad worked with a private structural engineering firm from eight to five, but then returned to work after having dinner with the family, on weeknights, to finish the day's work. My mom seemed to work from sunup to sundown, caring for the household as well as the four children and her parents who lived with us.

I know we don't get to choose our blood family, but as I reflect, I see what a significant role they had in shaping who I am today. I had many hours of "windshield time" in the car with Dad, and he was always my main cheerleader. He instilled in me early on that I could do anything I dreamed of and maybe even better than a boy. My mom always had the highest expectations of me, and she kept me motivated to work harder. My siblings were generally an annoyance, but they taught me a lot – not only how to fight and defend myself, but also how to share, problem-solve together, and how much fun it is to play together in those rare moments. I wouldn't trade it for the world.

As I look back, I now appreciate the stability of my family life. While growing up, there were set schedules, chores, and expectations, and everyone knew what had to be done for the day. With eight people living under one roof, it kept the chaos to a minimum, and life always had a regular order and rhythm. I now realize this was imperative for organizing my own life as an adult. It helped me develop my current lifestyle, and as I see my children become parents, I'm pleased to see this being passed on to their children.

The one thing that my parents and grandparents instilled in all of us kids was the value of education. This was a message we were repeatedly told, and we were expected to do our best in school. Our education was something no one could take away from us, and it was the key to a better future.

My family was not perfect; in fact, I now see that no family is perfect. However, there was an unspoken truth that bound us together forever. Despite our disagreements, we always knew that we had each other's backs, no matter what. My parents and grandparents have all passed on, but I've learned so many valuable things from them, and I, in turn, am trying to pass them on to my children and grandchildren.

The most valuable lesson I learned from my family was understanding what unconditional love meant. Similarly, our almighty God loves us, just as we are. Our imperfect human love is no match for God's perfect love. If we understand this, then we can start to live in a peaceful place, resting in His perfect love, even during these pandemic times. His love is characterized by grace and forgiveness, and it is eternal and unconditional!

> *"For it is by grace that you have been saved, through faith – and this is not from yourselves, it is the gift from God – not by your works, so that no one can boast."*

—EPHESIANS 2 8–10 NIV

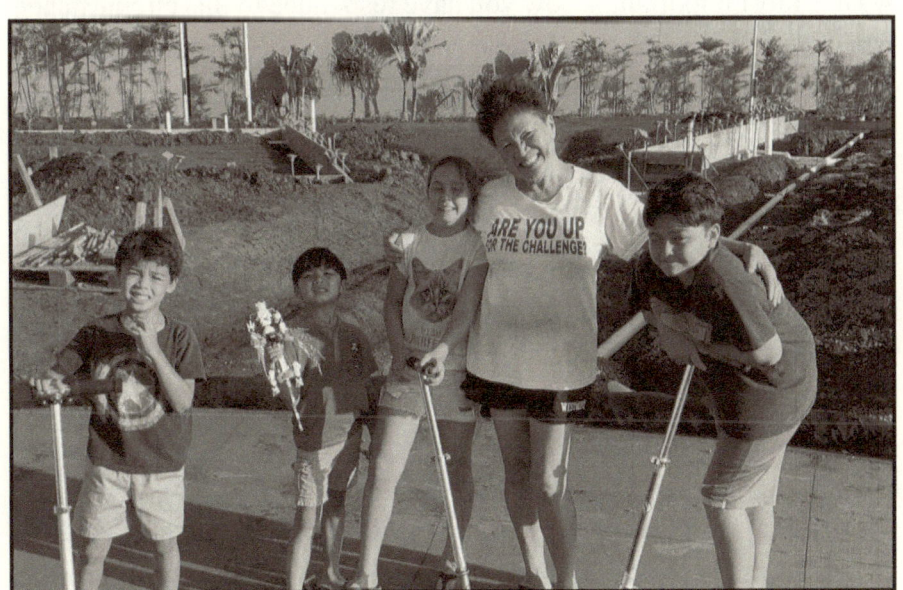

D ue to the COVID-19 pandemic, many traditions and gatherings have either been postponed or cancelled. Personally, it has affected me in several ways, including the postponement of funerals, weddings, graduations, trips, golf tournaments, and many more.

I want to share with you a very touching experience I had this past Sunday afternoon in Mililani. I heard cars honking and loud cheering coming from the main street. Martin and I got in the car, and to my surprise, I saw an entire community coming out on the streets to cheer for the graduating High School Senior class of 2020. It brought tears to my eyes to see the Aloha spirit in action.

I felt it was appropriate to offer a few parting words to this special 2020 class. I have secretly always wanted to give a commencement speech, so here is my version.

To the Class of 2020:

Across the world, graduates like you must leave behind the pomp and circumstance of graduation, but this does not lessen its significance or your achievement. You did not ask for this pandemic, but remember, what is most important is how you have responded to this circumstance, which will determine your character and success. Never stop dreaming big or working hard toward goals, no matter what others tell you. Adapt and be resilient, for now is your big opportunity to become that extraordinary person you were born to be.

I want to share with you a study that left a profound impact on me when my husband died ten years ago. It has been a guidepost on how I live my life today. I hope you can also learn something from this.

This study, conducted in 2010 by Rob Kelly, is entitled "Three Things Old People Wish They'd Done More of in Life." Here are his three surprising findings:

- *Leave a legacy.* Kelly defines legacy as "Anything handed down from the past, as from an ancestor or predecessor." In other words, leave a special gift to the generations that will follow you and know that you left this world a little better place.
- *Reflect more:* In this fast-paced world that we live in, there never seems to be time to pause and review the path of life we are on. It is vital that we take time out for ourselves and periodically revisit our priorities and life direction.
- *Take more risks:* There is a saying, "You don't regret what you did, only what you didn't do." Thus, in life, whether it is making decisions in relationships, career, hobbies, etc., choose to give it a try. Ask yourself, "What do I have to lose?" On your deathbed, you will be glad to know you lived a life of no regrets.

In conclusion, keep challenging yourselves and never stop learning. When you fall, as you inevitably will, get back up and continue to get back up. To the Class of 2020! Congrats and God bless!

"Listen to advice and accept discipline, and at the end you will be counted among the wise. Many are the plans in a person's heart, but it is the Lord's purpose that prevails."

—PROVERBS 19:20–21 NIV

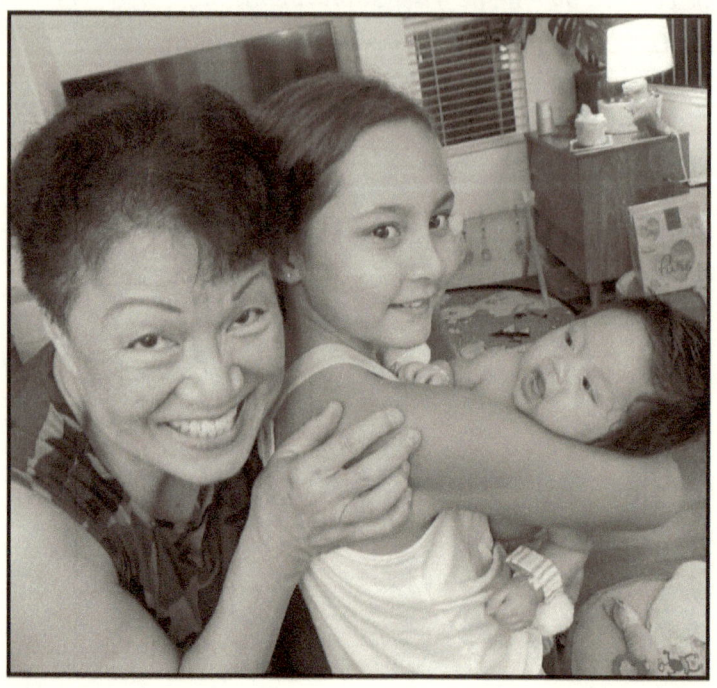

Today, I have been reading so many medical updates on how this pandemic is taking a toll on the mental health of our families, especially our children and teens. Recent stressors that have contributed to this toll include school closures, children at home, limited daycare and summer programs, parents losing their jobs, and food insecurity, among other factors. Experts now expect an increase in office and emergency room visits because of this elevated stress.

The recent buzzword in pediatrics right now is "ACE" or "Adverse Childhood Experiences," which makes this vulnerable population open to a lifetime of health concerns. "ACE," by definition, includes the following ten criteria: physical, emotional, and sexual abuse, physical and emotional neglect, growing up in a household where a parent was mentally ill, substance dependent, or incarcerated, parental separation or divorce, or domestic violence. The studies show that the more of these a child or teen has experienced, the greater the risk for lifelong physical, mental, and behavioral problems.

As pediatricians, we are now learning what to look for and actively reaching out to our patients to help them. Parents, if you feel that you're reaching your limit, it's understandable and it is okay, even necessary, to reach out for help. I hope that parents or guardians will realize that we, as their pediatricians, can be the bridge for them to access the necessary services or resources.

One recommendation to help remedy this situation is directed to those trusted adults who have a role in a child's life. This person could be a grandparent, aunt or uncle, coach, teacher, or church leader, and my advice to them is to spend a few minutes reaching out to that child, even if it is a simple text message or FaceTime chat. Sometimes, a small gesture like this can mean the world to a family under stress. It sends a message not only to the child, but also to the caregiver who may be struggling, that someone cares and, perhaps, they will know that they can reach out to you if the need arises.

I know that being a parent is highly stressful, but now with the added inconvenience of the COVID-19 pandemic lockdown, it is putting an even greater strain on families.

I want to reiterate that most primary care physicians' offices are still open, and it is safe to visit. We are taking the necessary precautions in our office to ensure a safe and sanitized environment for you. If you are still hesitant about coming in, consider a telehealth virtual visit with your physician.

So, dear reader, please help me spread the word about my deep concern for our children and families. Remind friends and family that there is no shame in seeking help. This can be done confidentially, and the sooner we can address any problems, the quicker we can come to a resolution.

Asking for help doesn't mean you're weak; it means you are strong and wise. Sometimes God helps us through other people. We must never be afraid to seek wise counsel and assistance from others.

"A wise son brings joy to his father, but a foolish man despises his mother. Folly brings joy to one who has no sense, but whoever has understanding keeps a straight course. Plans fail for lack of counsel, but with many advisers they succeed."

—PROVERBS 15:20–22 NIV

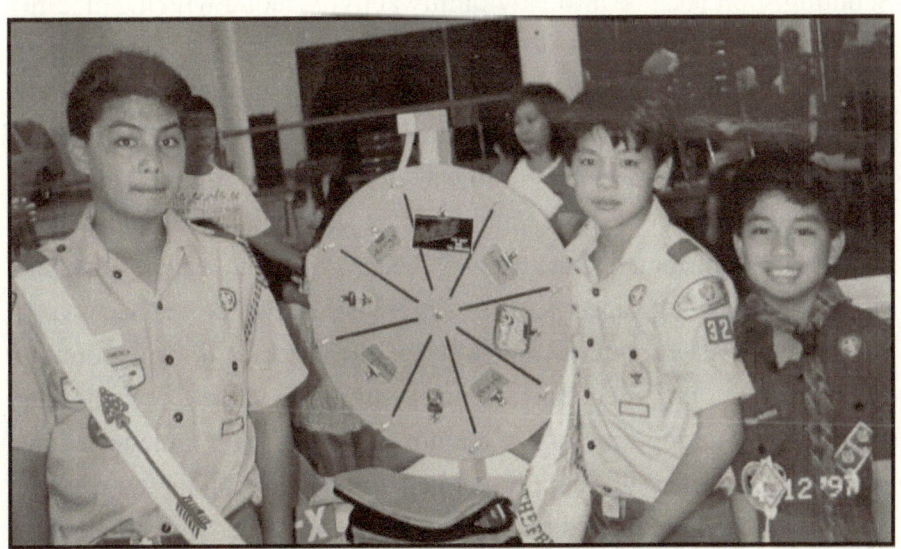

The COVID-19 pandemic has been truly difficult for families confined to their homes together for months, as I mentioned in my blog the other day. Families, like them or not, play a vital role in shaping who we are, our values, and the foundation from which we grow. Several years ago, there was a popular phrase, "It takes a village to raise a child," and what I have learned over the years is that the community we live in is also part of our extended family.

Today, I wanted to share with you how my Boy Scout family helped us in raising our four children (yes, even our daughter) into fine, productive citizens.

Back in the early 1990s, when our four children were all under ten years old, it was tough for us to enroll them in team sports due to our busy work schedules. However, right in the community where we lived, there was a young and rapidly growing Cub Scout Pack 167 and Boy Scout Troop 32. Our two older sons enrolled, and we soon found ourselves hosting weekly Cub Scout Pack meetings as well as occasional campouts in our backyard. Our youngest son and daughter also joined in the fun, and soon they were also participating in BB gun contests, light pole climbing competitions, fishing, hiking, and camping expeditions. Scouting soon became a weekly family activity, along with the monthly field trips with the entire Cub Scout Pack.

Probably the most rewarding part about Scouting was getting to know our neighbors and many other families in our tight-knit community of Gentry Waipio. We instantly became a "Scout Family" and had each other's backs. Just about every scouting parent, each with their unique skills and talents, contributed to the troop by becoming Scout leaders, planners, badge advancement supervisors, or simply helping wherever necessary.

We were all volunteers, but we worked together for one common goal: raising young men (and women) with good values. I recall many other leaders taking time out to mentor our sons. With three teen sons, we certainly needed this support and encouragement along the way.

Of course, there were times when we, as parents, as well as our sons, felt that Scouting was a chore, but I'm glad we all persevered. I think that we all learned many valuable life lessons. As young adults now, I see that these lessons learned are paying off well for them.

With sweat, hard work, and grit, all three of our boys achieved the rank of Eagle Scout, the highest level of achievement in Scouting. This was only possible through the help of the many caring people in my community, who came alongside us.

I continue to share my wonderful stories and memories of Scouting with other young families. Our children have learned to love God, their country, and the importance of loving one another through their Scouting experiences.

To my Scouting family: Thank you for being part of the "village" that helped us raise fine young adults. We are forever indebted to each of you who cared enough to volunteer time to Scouting.

> *"Two are better than one, because they have a good return for their labor: If either of them falls, one can help the other up. But pity anyone who falls and has no one to help them up."*

—ECCLESIASTES 4:9–10 NIV

This Memorial Day, we honor our brave service men and women who died while serving our country. I know I am incredibly grateful to all of them who made the ultimate sacrifice. As I've already mentioned, due to the current COVID-19 pandemic, many annual traditions and ceremonies in Hawaii have been cancelled, but our veterans are certainly not forgotten.

On this special day, let us also pause to remember our frontline healthcare and first responder heroes who put their lives on the line every day to care for all of us. Many lives have already been lost, and yet, they continue to show up to work daily to serve us. We salute all of you today and continue to pray for God's protection over you.

When our four children were growing up, we wanted them to remember how lucky they were to live in America and that many people sacrificed their lives for our freedom. Every Memorial Day, we had an annual tradition of going to the Punchbowl National Cemetery to place leis on each headstone. We did this activity with other Boy Scouts and found it was always well worth the time and effort.

My parents were both second-generation Chinese Americans who made many sacrifices for their families and their country. My dad joined the US Army the day after he turned eighteen. He then served at the Pearl

Harbor Naval Shipyard for the remainder of World War II. Dad loved his country so much that he would always sing patriotic songs to us. The words and melodies of these songs are committed to my memory to this day, and they always remind me of him.

My husband and I tried to instill similar values in our children. From a very young age, I wanted to give them a clear understanding of the duty and honor that come with being an American. My two older sons now work at Pearl Harbor Naval Shipyard, where they are keeping our submarines "fit to fight." My third son is a Captain in the Hawaii Air National Guard and works as an Air Battle Manager.

Today, dear readers, please take a moment to offer a prayer for all those who have made the ultimate sacrifice in service to our country and reflect on how blessed we are to live in the greatest nation in the world.

> *"My command is this: Love each other as I have loved you.*
> *Greater love has no one than this, than he lay down his life*
> *for his friends. You are my friends if you do what I command."*

—JOHN 15:12–14 NIV

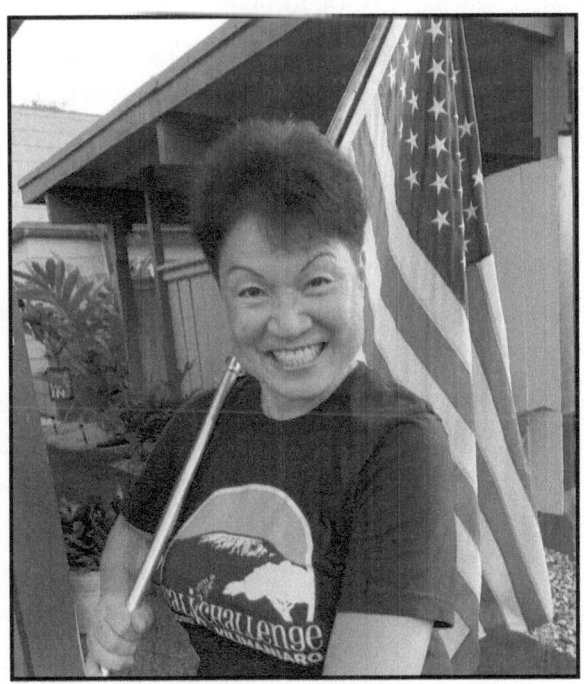

Today, I'll be honest. I was in a little bit of a "funk." I was thinking about going to the beach, but something always seemed to get in the way. So, it was back to our usual evening walks around the neighborhood. Don't get me wrong, it was fine, but sometimes, you feel like breaking the routine to do something different or have a change of scenery.

This past weekend, I did something I have been meaning to do for over five years. I ventured into a crowded Walmart and bought an American Flag kit. My wonderful husband immediately put it up. When the hardware was in place, he called for me to bring the fag out. As I walked out to the front with the flag, he was standing there, playing our National Anthem on his cell phone. We both sang the entire song and put the fag in place. This was such a sweet moment to remember.

Recently, something remarkable happened in Hawaii amidst the COVID-19 pandemic. An anonymous donor paid nearly 2,000 Seniors' groceries at Foodland Supermarket. This generous act came at a time when many people were in fear of going out, struggling to pay their bills, and dealing with social isolation, but this gesture meant more than just providing free groceries for these individuals. It sent a message of hope throughout our state. For me, it meant that there are still good people in the world, and anyone I encounter could be an excellent benefactor. We may never know who this benefactor is, but such a kind act will surely be remembered for a long time.

As I recall this story, I am reminded of similar stories I heard for the first time about my first husband at his funeral. Stephen was the President of our Gentry Waipio Community Association for many years, and he knew precisely which homes violated Association rules and were facing fines. He would often spend many lunch hours going to homes and making it right for them anonymously. I never knew he did any of this and thought he was going home to rest or nap. Some examples included helping a single mom fix her fence and mailbox or assisting an elderly couple with cutting down their weeds. When I think about these anonymous deeds, it brings tears to my eyes now, as it did then.

These anonymous acts of kindness warm my heart and restore my faith in humanity. There are, indeed, many good people out there who continue to do great things in a quiet, low-key manner, and they do it out of love for their fellow man.

So, dear readers, I encourage you to consider doing an anonymous good deed for someone you know or a stranger this week, knowing that you are generating more ripples of love in our world. We need this now.

> *"So, in everything, do to others what you would have them do to you, for this sums up the Law and the Prophets."*
>
> —MATTHEW 7:12 NIV

ENTRY: 05/27/20

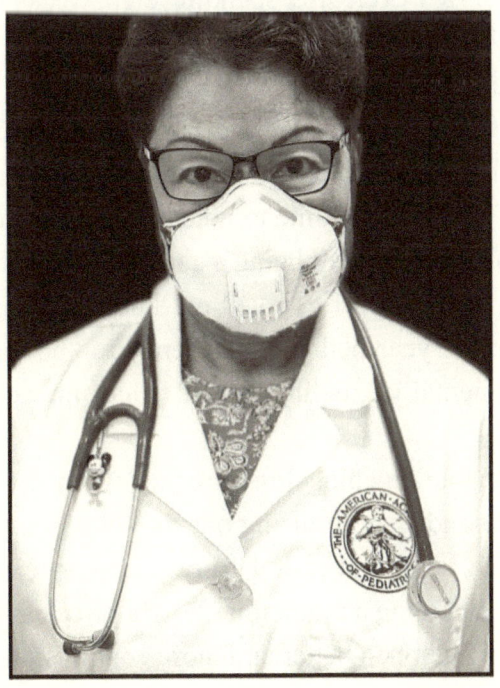

As the school year ends, I have been speaking with and listening to many of my graduating high school seniors in the office. They have had to miss their senior proms, awards banquets, graduation ceremonies, and other important events. However, to their credit, most of them have accepted their situation and look forward to their upcoming adventures. I have not heard one of them complain or whine. I am so very proud of them, and I let them know how I feel.

Today, I wanted to share with you, my dear readers, some of my thoughts on being a pediatrician. I feel I have a sacred job and duty to each one of my patients. Their parents have entrusted me to care for them – not only physically, but also in all other aspects of their lives.

When growing up, I loved playing with my siblings and the neighborhood kids. In high school, I spent many summers at the YMCA, first as a participant and then later as a volunteer Junior Leader. In college, I taught tennis in Nanakuli and assisted with the UH Freshmen Summer

Camps. As I started medical school, I was unsure of what specialty I wanted to pursue. However, after spending eight weeks in each specialty rotation in my third year, I quickly found my calling in Pediatrics, as it seemed a natural fit for me.

I will always be indebted to the patience and time my mentors invested in helping me gain invaluable knowledge and experience during my residency. They took the time to hold my hand and demonstrated to me, step by step, the "ropes" of being a good pediatrician. Many of them believed in me, even when I doubted my knowledge and competence. I compare my three-year pediatric residency to "boot camp" – It was physically and mentally grueling, but it taught me so much in just a short period.

Another valuable teaching lesson came when my husband and I began our family and started raising our four children. This experience taught me a great deal, and now I truly understand what my parents went through daily. Being a mother has been a priceless teaching lesson, and it has made me a much better and more compassionate pediatrician.

> *"At that time the disciples came to Jesus and asked, 'Who, then, is the greatest in the kingdom of God?' He called a little child to him and placed the child among them. And he said: 'Truly I tell you, unless you change and become like little children, you will never enter the kingdom of heaven. And whoever welcomes one such child in my name welcomes me.'"*
>
> —MATTHEW 18:1–5 NIV

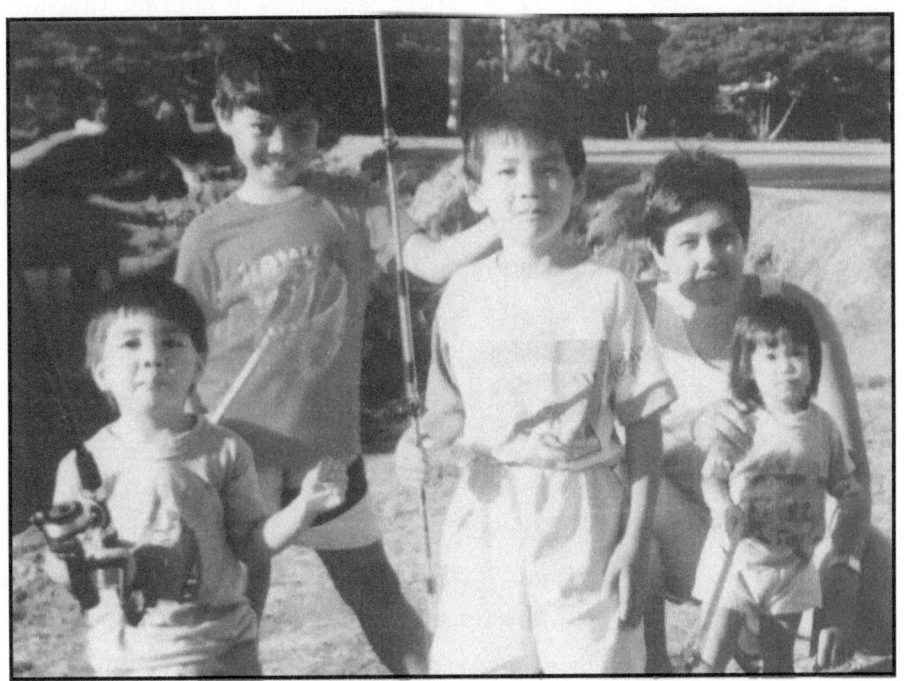

We are now over two months into the pandemic, and we are all wondering: When will this end? These are challenging times, and we all have many new things to learn. Daily routines have been completely disrupted, and we feel unbalanced.

Currently, one of the most important things to do is reestablish routines and regain control over our lives. As I see my families in the office, I hear how schedules have gone out the window. Routines are necessary to control chaos, and they have been proven, in the past, to improve not only your physical health but also your mental health.

Whenever we have any significant disruption in our lives, studies show that parenting patterns become less organized. This results in less discipline and fewer parent-child interactions during these times. The children, in turn, become upset, angry, aggressive, clingy, and anxious. They also start to regress, and this ultimately leads to more scolding, yelling, and punishments from the adults.

By maintaining routines after a significant disruption, children and teens feel reassured that they can expect continuity in their relationship with their parents, their most important bond. Here are some categories of routines to consider:

- Eat meals at regular times to provide a sense of security and maintain communication lines.
- Set a schedule for schooling, free play, exercise, and hygiene, even though you have the entire day at home. This will provide structure and more meaning for your day. Exercise and free play are essential routines and will directly help to reduce stress.
- Maintain the same bedtimes and routines, and ensure that the sleep times for naps, bedtime, and wake-up times remain as stable as possible. When everyone gets enough sleep, their mood stabilizes, and everyone feels less irritable.
- Chores should continue for all children, as it sends a message that life goes on as usual. It gives them a sense of control and a feeling of accomplishment in helping the family.
- Discipline should be maintained, and parents must expect children to continue to follow rules.

Finally, parents pause, sit quietly, and reflect on how they are feeling before reacting to a tense situation. This can be an excellent, teachable moment to share with your children. Don't forget that you are their role model, and they watch you every day. We must provide leadership to guide our child's behavior, attitudes, and beliefs, now and in the long term. Being a role model also means including your child in family discussions, living a healthy lifestyle, maintaining a positive attitude, taking responsibility for your actions, and more. We have an essential influence on our child's values and future choices, so the stronger the relationship with your child, the more impact you'll have.

"Listen, my son, to your father's instruction and do not forsake your mother's teaching. They are a garland to grace your head and a chain to adorn your neck. My son, if sinful men entice you, do not give in to them."

—PROVERBS 1 8–10 NIV

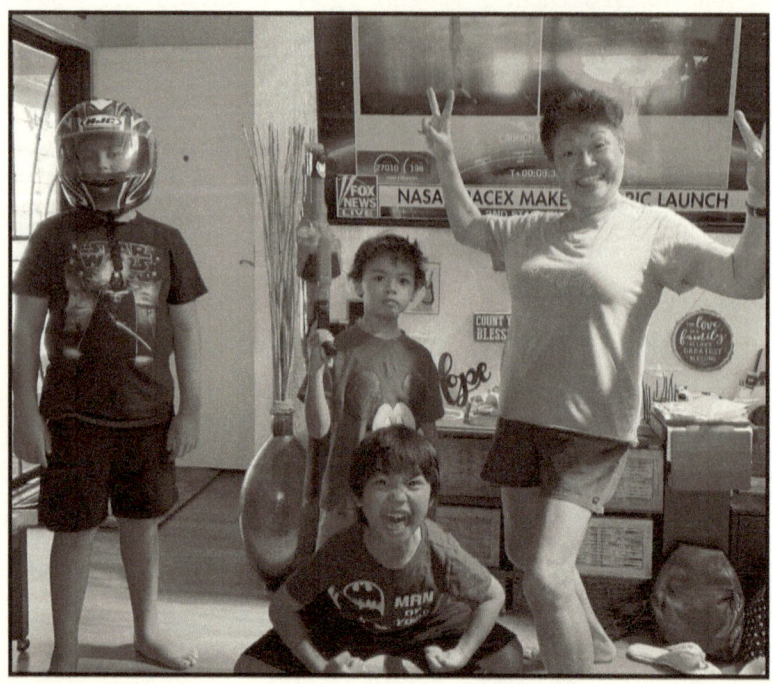

W ho said we can't have surprises during COVID-19 quarantine? This morning, we had a surprise visit from our three grandsons, and it was a welcome treat for Martin and me. I suggested we watch the historic launch of SpaceX's "Dragon" Rocket. This is the first time a private space transportation company has launched a vehicle into space to resupply the International Space Station. As we listened to the countdown, my husband came out wearing his motorcycle helmet, pretending to be an astronaut. Each of the boys screamed with delight, and they each had their turn wearing the helmet and pretending to be an astronaut in that spaceship. We have many precious photos to remember this moment.

This brought back fond memories of watching the Apollo 11 space mission in 1969. Our entire family watched our small, gritty television screen and screamed with excitement when astronaut Neil Armstrong came down the ladder and became the first person to walk on the moon.

He said these words that have stayed with me for my lifetime: "That's one step for man. One giant leap for mankind."

This moment was truly memorable, and I recall thinking how proud I was to be an American at that moment. Later, in my fourth year as a medical student in 1978, I remember seeing an ad recruiting women physicians to apply for NASA. For a moment, I thought about throwing in my application, but then I remembered how easily I get motion sickness.

"Lift up your eyes and look to the heavens: Who created all these? He who brings out the starry host one by one and calls forth each of them by name. Because of his great power and mighty strength, not one of them is missing."

—ISAIAH 40:26 NIV

4

JUNE

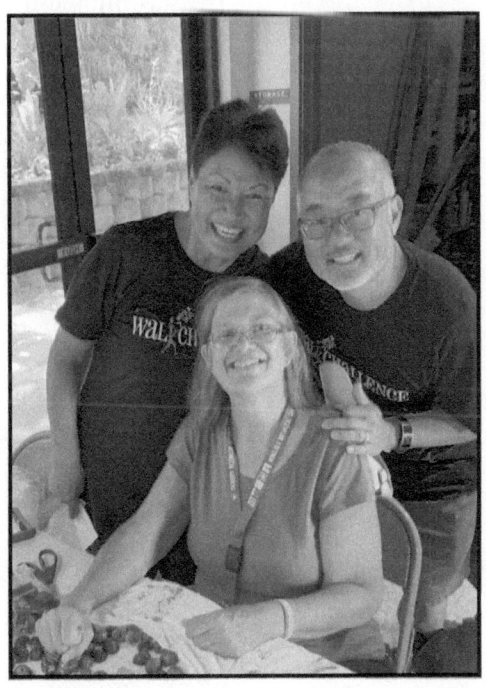

have been watching with much sorrow the continuing unrest occurring in our country. There have been live news reports of destruction and anger by the mobs at night, but then in the mornings, videos show people from these communities coming out to clean up. What a contrast. Stories like these give me hope and optimism for our nation. This reminds me of a saying: "The only thing necessary for evil to triumph is for good people to do nothing."

The question I have been thinking about is: *What can I do to help remedy this situation?* After much contemplation, I believe the answer lies within each of us. I believe everyone can make this world a better place. We can make a difference one person at a time, one day at a time, and one project at a time – and slowly, it will all add up to a lasting impact on the world.

To make a difference, you don't have to be brilliant, rich, or perfect; you must care about your fellow man and be present in the moment.

Once you decide to do something, you must not be afraid and take swift action. If we hesitate even for five seconds, our brains are wired to immediately come up with enough reasons why it's a bad idea. This procrastination then results in inaction.

So, perhaps at this time of COVID-19 and the awful killing of a man by a police officer, we must think about how we can act in the many lives we meet daily. Who knows, we could start positive ripples in someone's life by simply doing a small act of kindness. As I get older, I now know better and don't expect to see immediate results. However, if I were able to plant a seed of hope in someone's heart that could help them, then this would make me want to continue helping others.

Today, I wanted to share with you a personal story of hope that I continue to cherish. My friend's mom lost her husband, and she shared with me that her mom was having a tough time, even though it had been many years since his death. When I heard about this, I immediately wrote a letter to this woman, whom I had never met, and sent her a grief support book that has always given me great solace (*Healing after Loss* by Martha Whitmore Hickam). Several years passed, and I had completely forgotten about this event.

Recently, I finally got to meet my friend's mom when she came to visit her daughter in Hawaii. When I met her, she took an old, folded, and faded piece of paper from her wallet and read the letter I sent her many years ago. She told me she always kept it with her wherever she went because this gesture helped her decide to move forward in her life. This brought tears to my eyes when I heard this. The lesson I learned from this is that you never know how your actions will affect someone.

As a pediatrician, I never know how I am affecting children and their families. There are many days when I feel like no one is listening to me... but I plod along doing the best I can. I feel a deep obligation to the parents who have chosen me as their pediatrician and entrusted me with their precious children. Occasionally, patients and their families return with heartwarming stories of how my advice or treatment has helped them. These small, inspirational stories of gratitude always make me happy and reminds me of why I chose to pursue a career in medicine in the first place.

So, dear readers, there are two lessons to take home today. The first is to let your physician know if they made a difference in your life, as we are only human and sometimes need to hear some positive feedback. The second lesson can be summed up in words by Nelson Mandela, "We can all change the world and make it a better place. It is in our hands to make a difference."

I believe that God has a great plan for each of you, so step forward, reach out, and help each other today.

> *"Heal me, O Lord, and I shall be healed; save me and I will be saved, for you are the one I praise."*

> —JEREMIAH 17:14 NIV

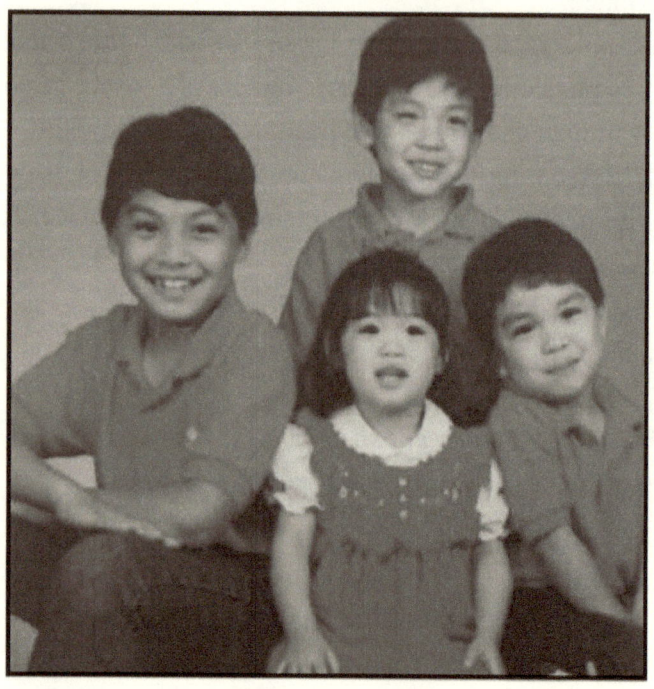

Hello, dear readers, I hope you are all being "safer at home." I am still waiting to see when we can come together in groups of over ten. I continue to see patients in my office, and parents are slowly bringing their children back in for their well exams and vaccines. Due to the pandemic's "safer at home" rule, and with families being cooped up at home, I have been seeing more families coming in where the children have taken over the house. Parents are tired, and they tell me that they want some peace. Thus, they are allowing their children to do whatever they please. The children stay up late playing video games or watching television, and eating anything at any time, forgetting all chores, and even being disrespectful to the adults.

This is the prevailing snapshot of many families right now, where it's easier and more convenient to take the easy route by allowing the kids to do whatever they want. As a parent, I understand that we never want to see our child crying or in distress, but doing this will lead to dire consequences. Growing up means everyone must face challenges, be self-sufficient, and respect authority. The sooner children learn these coping skills, the better they will be in the long run. When children are not taught to be independent or have good coping skills, they soon become young adults with a lifelong cycle of dependence and anxiety.

Currently, the most common childhood psychiatric problems are anxiety disorders. Children with these diagnoses are miserable and constantly frightened, worried, or physically ill due to their anxiety. They have difficulties in academics as well as fitting in and making friends. Their parents witness this distress daily, feel a great deal of guilt, and then quickly act to make their kids happy again by giving in to their demands.

For myself, when growing up, none of the adults in my life "gave in" to us kids. We each had chores to do every day. I grew up in a household of eight people, and there was always an abundance of things to do. We never got any allowance, but we just did chores because if we didn't, there would be consequences. Sure, I didn't like or agree with all the rules my parents implemented, but I always knew they were fair and in place to keep us four kids in line. We were also expected to have the utmost respect for our grandparents, parents, teachers, and other authority figures. Having a good understanding of this concept later served me well in both school and life.

I feel the current problem in parenting these days is that well-meaning parents are unknowingly getting sucked into the cycle of anxiety. They give in to their children too soon and allow them to escape many challenging situations that could have taught them life lessons. Over time, these children develop into young adults who become increasingly anxious and lack confidence in themselves. As a result, we now have young adults living at home with their parents who are not working, have no meaningful relationships, or purpose in life.

Considering all of this, I advocate that we adopt parenting styles that prioritize love for our children, while also teaching them to respect authority and stand on their own two feet from the outset. It is imperative that they learn that they are not the center of the universe, need to become independent, and understand that their parents are not always going to be at their "beck and call." It is only then that our youth can grow up into happy, productive, and confident adults. And boy, does our world need this more than ever now.

> *"Fathers, do not exasperate your children; instead, bring them up in the training and instruction of the Lord."*
>
> —EPHESIANS 6:4 NIV

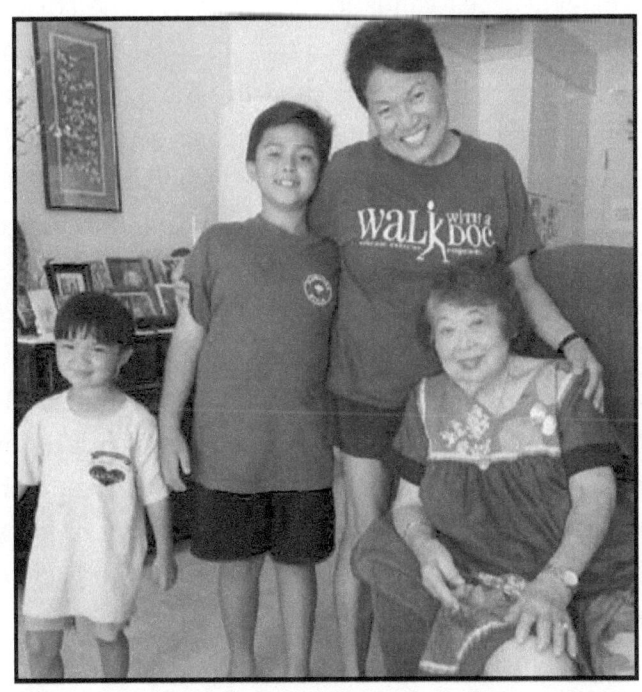

During this pandemic, Martin and I have continued to walk nearly every evening for the past three months. Along the way, we always see neighbors, friends, and former patients or their parents. This past week, someone stopped me and told me how grateful she was to me for being her grandson's pediatrician. She raised him as her son, and he is now in the Air Force. This was a brief encounter, but it meant a great deal to me. I genuinely appreciate times when people tell me that I made even a slight difference in their child's life.

Sadly, I have been to many funerals where people tell stories about how that person impacted their lives after they have passed. Dear readers, the time to express your gratitude to someone is now. You never know how long this person will be around, and if you wait for the "next time," it might be too late. Not only will it make you and the person feel good, but it will also validate someone who mattered to you and encourage them to continue reaching out to others.

I believe that everyone, regardless of age, gender, occupation, race, or religious belief, needs validation that they matter. There are many people I have cherished and admired over the years. They are the ones who believed in me and took the time to mentor me. Through their reassuring words and actions, they guided me on my journey toward accomplishing my goals. I have always tried to tell each of these important people that I am so grateful for all they have done for me, many times. As I grow older, they have been my role models, and I only hope that I am paying it forward, just as they did, to other young people.

In my own life, I strive to acknowledge everyone I encounter daily and let them know that they are valued and matter. It could be the cashier, waitress, co-workers, family, or friends, and all it takes is a simple smile or a greeting like "good morning" as you pass them. Additionally, I've learned how important it is to listen to them when we are in a conversation entirely. Mr. Rogers got it right when he said, "More and more, I've come to understand that listening is one of the most important gifts we can do for one another."

It is only when we are fully present that others will feel like the center of our attention and know that they matter to us. It only takes a few minutes of investment, but this investment in them will go a long way.

Continue to keep in mind that mattering is a choice. We are not obligated to do this, but what a better world this would be if we all thought like this.

So, this is my homework for each of you this week: Take every opportunity to let others know that they matter. It doesn't matter how you do it; you can tell them in person, write a note, or make a call. However, you do it, choose to advise, offer, encourage, thank, inspire, or inform them that you notice them and believe in them. It won't take much effort on your part, but I know it will make a world of difference in their lives.

God has a plan for everyone, and you can be the one who influences one person, who in turn influences two more people, and so forth. Always place your trust in the Lord and know that, even in our small actions, we can all contribute to making the world a better place.

"Let us hold unswervingly to the hope we profess, for he who promised is faithful. And let us consider how we may spur one another on toward love and good deeds. Let us not give up meeting together, as some are in the habit of doing, but let us encourage one another, and all the more as you see the Day approaching."

—HEBREWS 10:23–25 NIV

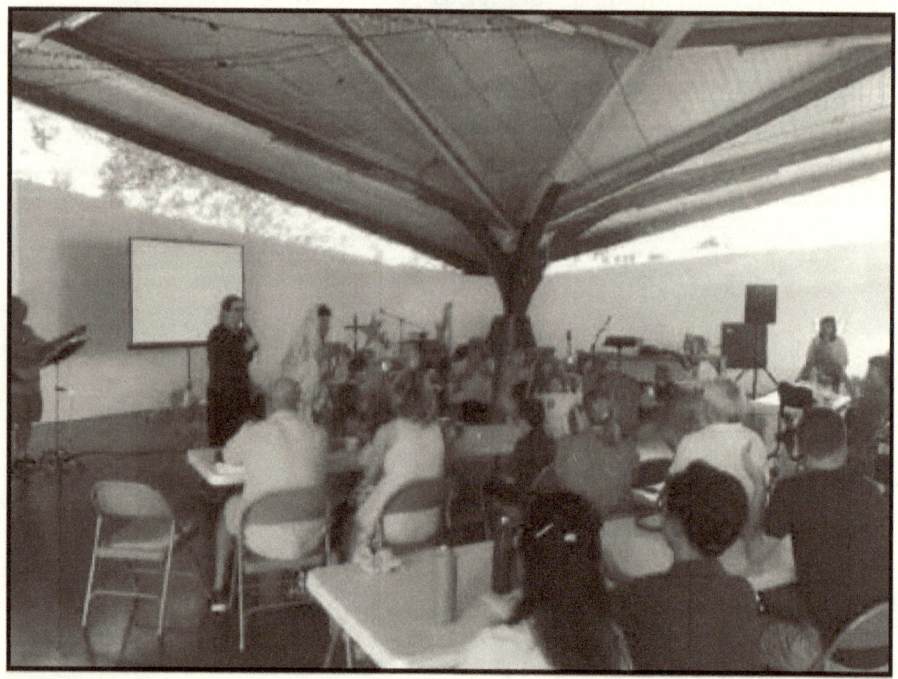

Yesterday's in-person Sunday church service was such a blessing for me. This was the first time we had met in person in months, since the COVID-19 lockdown began. It felt great to see everyone in person once again. This was precisely what I needed.

My wonderful church, Momilani Christian Church, in Pearl City, is an intimate one with approximately twenty-five members. Pastor Jerry Higashi has been incredibly encouraging during these pandemic times, consistently pointing us back to the Bible to find our answers. These are the exact times when we need to go back to the source, God, rather than assume the truth is in the televised news commentaries or what's written on social media.

Pastor Jerry's sermon focused on what Christians can do to be part of the solution. He put out a call to action and told us to join the "revolution" to love one another, proclaim God's love, and return to the Ten Commandments.

I believe that the slow deterioration of our country is our own doing. By keeping God out of our homes, schools, workplaces, and other public spaces, we have lost our way and no longer know the truth. We now know of many examples where Christians are deliberately being singled out and persecuted. But God never said it would be easy to stand up for Him, and this is precisely what we all need to be doing now.

I want to be a part of this "revolution," but what can one person do for the "revolution?" The way I see it is, it must start somewhere, so why not me? This means I'll be intentional about reaching out to others I encounter daily. I'll share as much as I can about the message of God's love, hope, and plan for each one of us.

On another note, I had a benchmark day on Saturday when I received two vital pieces of mail that I had been waiting for. I received my first shipment of printed books, The Happy, Healthy Revolution: A Working Parent's Guide to Achieving *Wellness as a Family Unit,* as well as my Medicare Part A membership card. I was so excited that I asked Martin to take a photo of this moment.

I'll be sixty-six years old in August, and I am proud of my Medicare card. I don't know how I've reached this age, but it is my badge of wisdom and experience. As my kids tell me, I'm reaching my twilight years, but I hope God gives me many more years to continue His work on this Earth.

> *"Now this is eternal life: that they may know you, the only true God, and Jesus Christ, whom you have sent. I have brought you glory on earth by completing the work you gave me to do. And now, Father, glorify me in your presence with the glory I had with you before the world began."*
>
> —JOHN 17:3–5 NIV

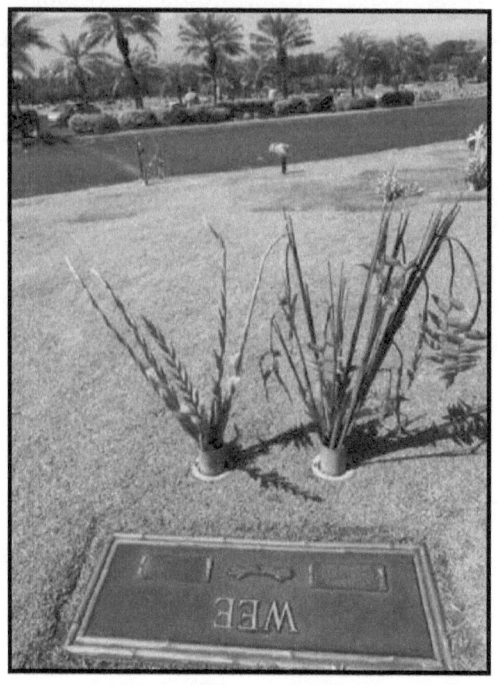

On this day, ten years ago, my husband of thirty years died suddenly and unexpectedly. When Stephen passed away suddenly, I was utterly blown away by the outpouring of kindness from the entire community. On the day of the funeral, Thursday, July 1, people were already standing in line one or two hours before the viewing time. We were anticipating many people, but the sheer numbers that came to pay their respects were overwhelming. The line circled the building, and it seemed as though the entire community had come out to say goodbye to Stephen.

After the funeral, our family opened over 600 sympathy cards, and the expressions of love and what Stephen meant to them helped get me through those first few months. I want to thank each of you for helping me through this difficult time in my life. Mahalo! You were all my angels.

I still don't understand why God took Stephen home at such a young age, but only He sees the big plan for each of us. Today, I will look up to Heaven and thank Him for the time we had together and all He has done and continues to do to sustain me.

So, dear readers, I leave you with a remembrance of Stephen, which is the dedication of my first book:

> "For Stephen L. Wee, MD…. You are so loved and so missed, but your legacy of compassion and service to others lives on. Thank you for being such a wonderful husband, father, and physician. You have positively touched and changed so many lives in your brief lifetime."

> *"Now, when he saw the crowds, he went up to the mountainside and sat down. His disciples came to him, and he began to teach them, saying: 'Blessed are the poor in spirit, for theirs is the kingdom of heaven. Blessed are those who mourn, for they will be comforted.'"*

> —MATTHEW 5:1–4 NIV

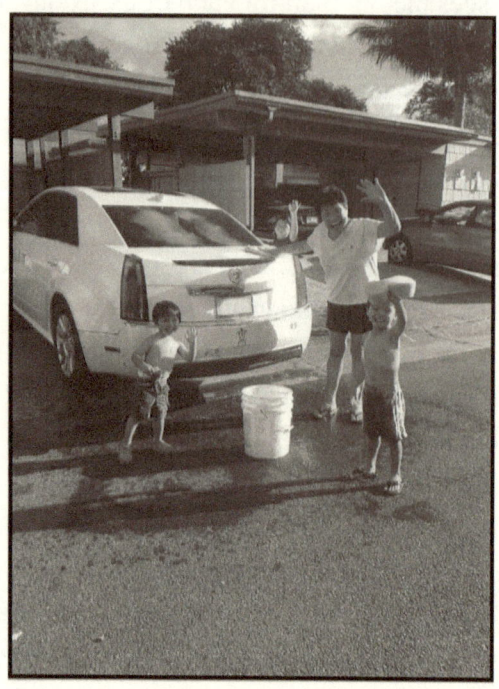

Saturday has finally arrived, and I encourage everyone to go outdoors and enjoy the world's most beautiful weather. Simply spending time outdoors has numerous positive benefits, as I've already mentioned, but one of the most important benefits is that it has a "de-stressing" effect. I believe we are all in need of this right now.

We're still dealing with COVID-19, as well as the recent chaos and rioting that have been seen in our nation. I want to be informed about timely events, but there have been times when I have had to turn away from the news and walk away. I sometimes feel very frustrated with everything going on around me.

Today, our Governor extended the two-week quarantine for visitors to Hawaii until the end of July. I'm not sure if this is the right call in our already devastated tourism economy, but on the other hand, we don't want visitors to bring the COVID-19 virus to Hawaii, causing a second wave.

I wanted to remind everyone that you can control your stress response. It is essential to do this because stress itself puts all of us at increased risk for even more physical and mental health problems. Some of these include decreased metabolism and weight gain, muscle and joint pains, gastrointestinal problems, decreased immune system, and the worsening of any pre-existing mental illness. Managing stress well helps us to live healthier, happier, and more productive lives.

Here are some tips to help you control the stress in your life:

- Tip 1: Identify the sources of stress in your lives. Keeping a daily stress journal can help you identify the sources of stress.
- Tip 2: Practice the 4 As of stress management:

Avoid: learn to say no and steer clear of people or environments that cause you stress.
Alter: Express your feelings and be open to compromising.
Adapt: Look at the big picture and reframe the problem.
Accept: Let go of things you cannot change and learn to forgive.

Tip 3: Increase your physical activity by walking as many steps as possible each day.
Tip 4: Connect to others virtually, by phone or write a letter.
Tip 5: Schedule time for fun and relaxation; otherwise, it will never happen.
Tip 6: Adopt a healthy lifestyle by eating more vegetables/ fruits, reducing processed foods and sugar intake, and getting enough sleep.
Tip 7: Spend time daily meditating.

Finally, during these stressful times, it's good to remember that God is always there to help us. He is watching over us, and all we must do is ask for His help.

"Come to me, all who labor and are heavily laden, and I will give you rest. Take my yoke upon you, and learn from me, for I am gentle and lowly in heart, and you will find rest for your souls. For my yoke is easy, and my burden is light."

—MATTHEW 11:28

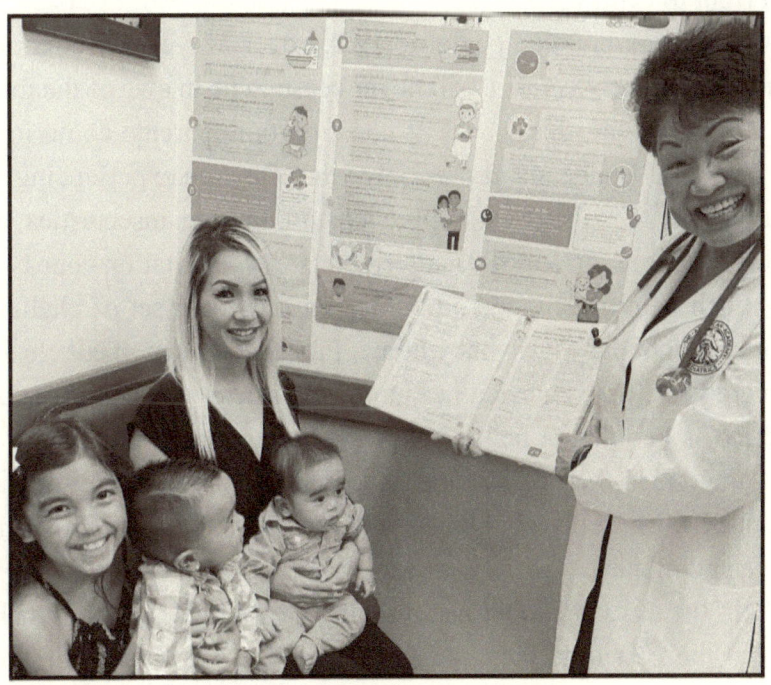

L ast night, I attended a small family baby shower for my granddaughter, Karter, who is expected to arrive in a few weeks. This will be our fifth grandchild, and I'm eager to meet her.

Beginnings are always so beautiful, exciting, happy, and full of hope. Attending the baby shower reminded me of the time I was pregnant with my first baby, as a newly trained pediatric resident. You would think I had complete confidence in being a new mom, but all I could think of were the worst scenarios. Perhaps my training at a large tertiary children's hospital conditioned me to feel this way and made me prepared for the worst. In my three years of residency training, I had already seen so much death, pain, and suffering in children of all ages.

As I approached my due date, my mentor and dear friend, Dr. Annemarie Sommer, whom I had already mentioned, looked me directly in the eyes and said, "Everything is going to be okay, and I'll be there with you." This is precisely what I needed, and indeed, everything went well. Sometimes, all it takes is a simple affirmation that everything will be all right to calm you down.

As a private practice pediatrician for over 35 years, I continue to see newborns every week. I will never cease to be in awe of the miracle of a new birth into this world. When first-time parents come in with their newborn, I understand precisely what they are experiencing. That first night home is filled with apprehension, fatigue, insecurities, and a million questions. It doesn't matter if this is your first or your twelfth baby. Each baby is unique and comes with its own set of challenges. When I brought our fourth baby home, I recalled this moment clearly as if it were yesterday. I carried her in, set the carrier down, and sat down and cried as I could not believe we were doing this all over again. Why would anyone in their right mind have babies…. They are a significant amount of work, rob you of sleep, and require a substantial investment of time and money.

Well, the answer is obvious. Ask any new parent, and they will tell you that the first time they see their little one, it's love at first sight. Your world suddenly expands, and now it's not only about you, but also about your family and their future. As a new mom, I began to look at life differently, and the entire future seemed brighter and more exciting. I had great hopes for my child's future, and I wanted to be the best parent I could be, whatever that looked like.

As I continue to see patients in my office, I especially enjoy doing the final eighteen-year physical exams on the patients I've cared for since they were newborns. I am always in disbelief when I see my "babies" suddenly all grown up now. I'm reminded once again how quickly time. flies. I always try to send them off with some profound, sage advice, such as calling your mom once a week, eating your veggies and fruits, getting enough sleep… but most of all, pursuing your dreams and never, ever giving up.

I will miss them, and I can only hope that I have done the best I could as their pediatrician. It is refreshing to see them grow into fine young men and women in our community, working and starting families of their own. I am even beginning to see the second generation of children from those first patients.

Some parents say that I am a "strict" physician, but I'd like to say that I am passionate about my work and care deeply about helping each child reach their fullest potential, which is what God created them to be. I genuinely believe we all have a unique purpose in this world, and it takes a village to help our youth succeed, because, as I see it, they are our future.

I love my job, and I love my families. I try to be that voice for the "voiceless," and I thank God for the privilege of being a pediatrician. Parenting is perhaps the most challenging job God has given to us, but if we look to God and the Bible, He promises to provide us with all that we need.

> *"Unless the Lord builds the house, its builders labor in vain. Unless the Lord watches over the city, the guards stand guard in vain. In vain you rise early and stay up late, toiling for food to eat – for he grants sleep to those he loves. Children are a heritage from the Lord, offspring a reward from him."*
>
> —PSALM 127:1–3 NIV

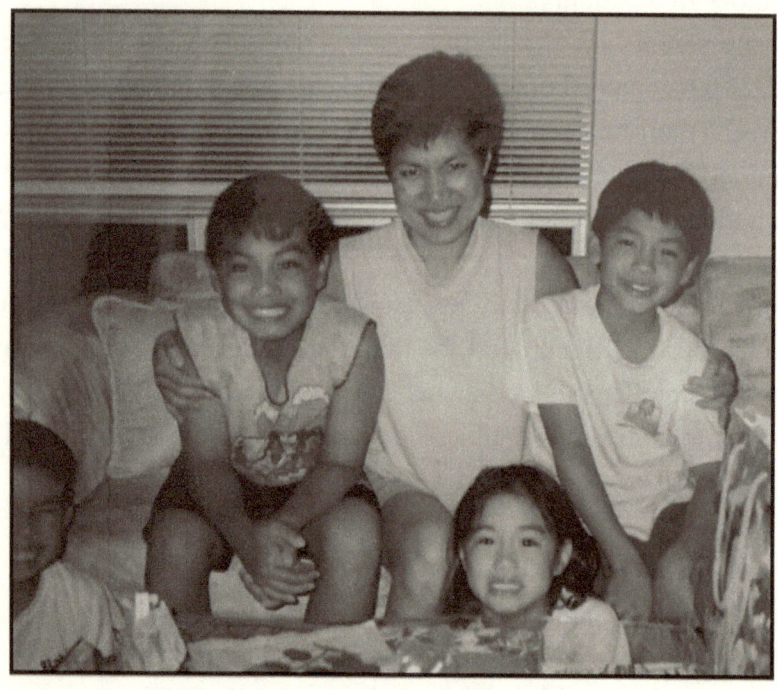

always look forward to Sundays, as it replenishes my soul each time. It felt great to be back with my church family in person yesterday. We had sixteen members attend, and it was wonderful to gather, worship, and pray together.

Today, after church, I had the opportunity to have lunch with my oldest son, daughter-in-law, and three grandsons. It was lovely to hug them and spend some quality time together in person. This pandemic has caused many of us to become socially isolated, and somehow, Face Timing just isn't the same.

So today, I wanted to discuss the importance of family units. Parents are the first relationship and experiences for our children. It's essential to offer a safe, stable, and nurturing environment from birth. During these uncertain times, with families in lockdown, this becomes an even more important topic to discuss, as a strong unit will help us immensely as we navigate our way through these times.

As a pediatrician, I have witnessed the gradual erosion of the family over the past three decades. I started very naïve but soon realized the enormous impact of family discord. I have, therefore, made it my mission not only to be a physician for my patients, but also an ardent advocate for parents. If the family unit is strengthened, the child's health and well-being are more likely to be secure.

Parents are the backbone of the family, and at each visit, I make it a point to discuss maintaining healthy parental authority. From my observation, children often benefit when you are not their "best friend forever." They will only prosper and succeed if they see parents working together and enforcing consistent rules and schedules. If you ask any parent, this is probably one of the hardest things to do, but the benefits will far outweigh any discomfort or time invested. I occasionally encounter parents who disagree with my parenting style, and this results in even more confusion and chaos. Parents need to come together as a team. In situations where this is difficult, marriage counseling has helped save marriages and families. When a strong, loving relationship exists between a husband and wife, it sets an excellent example for their children, who will become the parents of tomorrow.

At many well-child visits, I often turn to the new dad and ask him, "When was the last time you took your wife out for a date?" The sleepy-eyed parents always look shocked, and I know that's the last thing on their mind. However, as a seasoned mother myself, I recall my husband and me making a vow always to have two dates a week. This was such a saving grace for our marriage, and I always looked forward to my "dates" with my husband to check in with one another and rekindle the flame of romance.

> *"Submit to one another out of reverence for Christ. Wives, submit to your own husbands as to the Lord. For the husband is the head of the wife as Christ is the head of the church, his body, of which he is the Savior. Now as the church submits to Christ,*

so also wives should submit to their husbands in everything.
Husbands, love your wives just as Christ loved the church and
gave himself for her."

—EPHESIANS 5:21–25 NIV

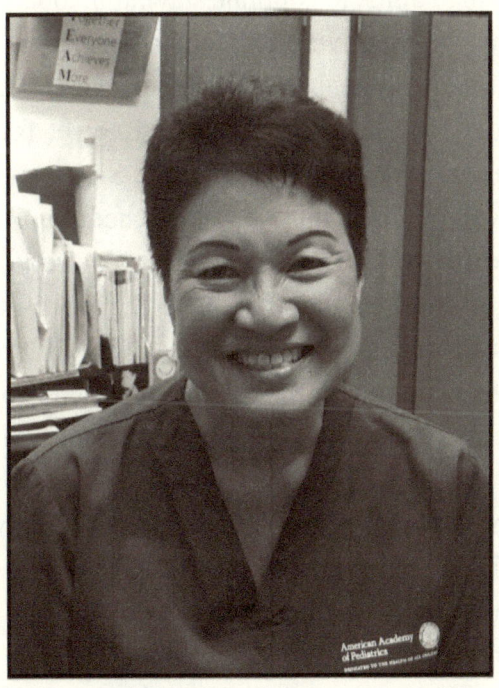

A s I watch local and national news, I feel we are constantly fed conflicting messages. On the one hand, they report that COVID-19 pandemic cases are decreasing, and then the next day, they report a spike. With all this constant uncertainty and fear around us, it can sometimes be challenging to remain calm. Our children are constantly watching our reactions, so we must take the time to reassure them. This could be as simple as telling them that you will always be there for them and assuring them that the entire family will get through this period.

I tell parents it is okay to address their fears honestly and, in an age-appropriate way. They are hearing the same frightening news that you and I hear, so they need help understanding its impact on them. Continue to remind them that handwashing, social distancing, and staying at home is essential to help everyone remain safe.

When children start to act up, acknowledge their feelings calmly and tell them you understand they're upset because their friends cannot come over, or that they are confined to home. Suggest ways for everyone, including adults, to continue staying in touch with family and friends via phone, email, or virtual meetings on Zoom.

Once again, maintain healthy routines for the entire family to keep the home in order. The days should have time set for meals, snacks, schoolwork, chores, exercise, and free time. Sit down as a family and get everyone involved in planning out this schedule.

During these stressful times, it's natural for everyone to be a little anxious. Younger children may not have the words to express their feelings, and, as a result, they may act out. Older children may become irritable due to missing out on time with their friends or attending special events. Parents can try to redirect bad behavior by replacing it with family activities, such as a hike, bike ride, art project, or gardening.

Another important reminder is for parents and caregivers to acknowledge and reward good behaviors. This is not as easy as it sounds, because as parents, we are often conditioned to notice only negative behaviors. If your child is not engaging in behavior that could harm themselves or others, rewarding good behavior and ignoring bad behavior can be an effective way to stop it.

Finally, parents, be sure to take care of yourselves and get enough sleep. Find ways to take some breaks throughout the day, and if the other parent is at home, take turns watching the children.

> *"Not only so, but we also glory in our sufferings, because we know that suffering produces perseverance; perseverance, character; and character, hope. And hope does not put us to shame, because God's love is poured out into our hearts through the Holy Spirit, who has been given to us."*
>
> —ROMANS 5:3–5 NIV

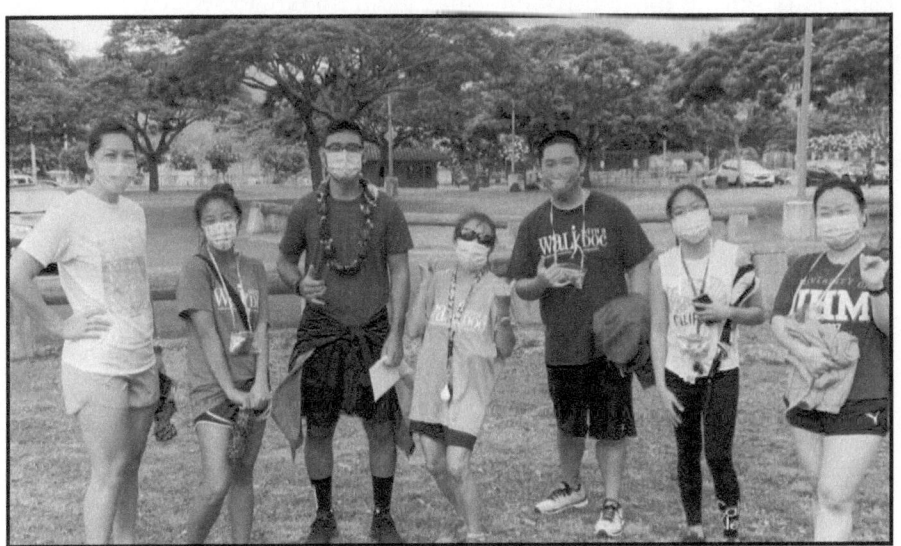

Today's blog was suggested by my husband, Martin. When we go walking every evening, it is a fantastic way for us to catch up on how our day went. I recently shared with him some heartwarming answers to a question I ask every patient at their well-visit checkup. That question is: "What are you going to be when you grow up?" Martin always enjoys hearing their answers, and he suggested I share them with you, so here they are.

I love to ask this question because I believe it is beneficial for everyone, regardless of age, to reflect on their future goals and life's purpose. I think it is never too early to consider the many possibilities.

As a little girl, I was fascinated by biographies, especially those of famous women. After reading the biography of Dr. Elizabeth Blackwell, the first woman doctor, I announced to my family at the tender age of eight that I wanted to be a doctor, just like her. Back in the sixties, there were very few women doctors in Hawaii, but that did not stop me from dreaming of this. I recall many times well-meaning adults telling me that becoming a nurse would be a more suitable career choice. The only person who truly believed in me from the start was my dad, and he never wavered in his faith in me. That was all I needed to push me through, especially during those difficult times along the journey.

Recently, a three-year-old boy responded to my question without hesitation, stating that he wanted to be Optimus Prime, a large Transformer monster truck. Hey, please don't laugh; he got an answer and gave it. A four-year-old girl told me right away that she wanted "to be bigger." Many children have a new answer for me each year, and some don't have the faintest clue of what they want to be for many years. I have also encountered many who consistently provide me with a response each year, and I strive to be the person who affirms them annually.

I have always been a firm believer that God has given each person a unique set of talents and abilities, and He has a definite purpose for them to discover and pursue. Sometimes, I'll try to point out my patient's strengths and encourage them to actively think about how they can take this information to help them decide what they would like to do when they grow up.

Many years ago, I had a seven-year-old boy who immediately answered my question and said he wanted to be a neurosurgeon. He even knew correctly what this physician did. He is now graduating from medical school and will be entering a neurosurgery residency in St. Louis, Missouri.

There was another patient who had over a hundred febrile seizures during his childhood years. His parents were always concerned, but I kept reassuring them that he would be fine. The family relocated to the mainland many years ago, and I recently received a text from his mom. She wrote that he was now attending medical school. She shared an essay in which he wrote that I was his inspiration to become a physician, which touched me deeply.

For the past several weeks, I have encountered three young women, high school graduates, who told me their goal was to be a pediatrician. Medicine is not an easy field, but the rewards are great. I'm happy to help and encourage young men and women to consider this career.

The lesson I want to share with you today is to encourage our youth to dream big and dare to imagine all the possibilities that lie ahead for them. We must give them words of affirmation because it only takes one person to believe in them.

During this season of graduation and new transitions, let's all take the opportunity to encourage our youth to explore and pursue their life's purpose, for which God created them.

> *"Remember your leaders, who spoke the word of God to you.*
> *Consider the outcome of their way of life and imitate their faith.*
> *Jesus Christ is the same yesterday and today and forever."*

—HEBREWS 13:7–8 NIV

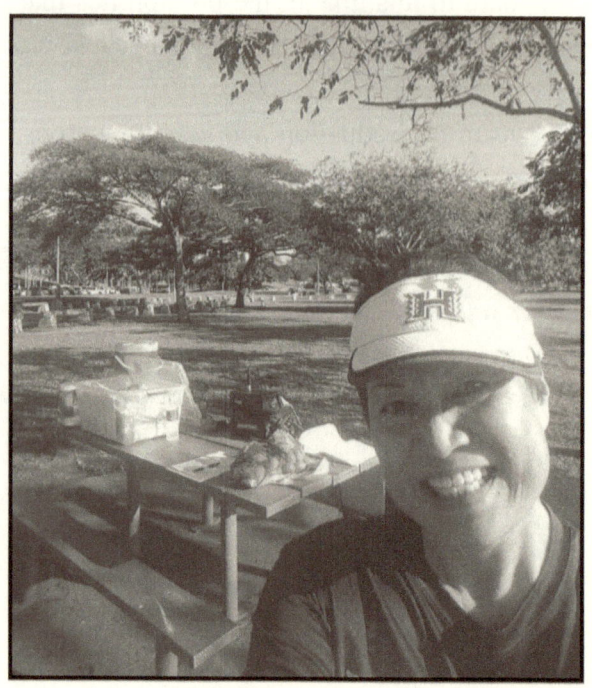

Today is Father's Day, and I feel saddened that I cannot be with my children to celebrate this special day. We would have gotten together and had dinner to remember Dad as well as celebrate my two older sons' fatherhood. I visited both to drop a card and a small Father's Day present. I am so proud to see the amazing fathers they have become, and I know, in large part, they had a great role model.

As I am sitting here today, I cannot help but remember my dad, who passed away in 2003. His parents arrived in Hawaii from China, seeking a better life. Dad was born in Honolulu and had five siblings. They all worked at their small, "Mom and Pop" general store in Kalihi, located on Palama Street. My paternal grandfather was a "Manapua man" who would go out each morning with two baskets hanging from a pole on each side of him and sell his sweet pork buns and other snacks.

Dad always told me that his parents encouraged him to get a good education, as they know it was the key to success. Dad attended Catholic schools and excelled in math and science.

The day after my dad turned eighteen, he volunteered for the US Army and was stationed at the Pearl Harbor Naval Shipyard, where he performed desk duties. Within a few months, the war ended, and my dad never got to see front-line action. However, he decided to use the GI Bill to further his education. I'm always amazed to think of where my dad chose to go. He decided to attend the Massachusetts Institute of Technology and spent five years in Boston to attain his master's degree in Structural Engineering. Whether he was in Boston or not, he met my mom, also a Hawaii resident, who earned her master's degree in social work at Boston University. They met, got married, and returned to Hawaii to raise our four children.

What I loved the most about my dad was his giving heart. We had people visit us on weekends to seek his advice on their taxes, various projects, or to share stories. He also helped family and friends, at a moment's notice, with their immigration papers or any other matters whenever he could. He performed many acts of kindness quietly, humbly, and without much fanfare.

Dad was probably my biggest fan in my pursuit of being a doctor. He never once wavered in his support for me. During the sixties, he was the only person who truly believed in me and all I needed to do was keep pushing forward. We used to have many discussions about life and other deep philosophical topics.

The most important thing he shared with me was his deep belief in God and the power of trusting Him in all things. Of course, along my journey, many other mentors came alongside me at just the right time, but Dad was there for the entire journey. As I look back, I realize that every person in my life was placed there by God, and I know for a fact that these were not coincidences.

I did not arrive at where I am today by myself, and I can only hope that I'm doing as good a job of "paying it forward" to other young men and women who cross my path.

During this pandemic, I'm thinking about how lucky I was to have you for my dad. Thank you, Dad, for your love, unwavering support, and belief in me. I couldn't have done it without you, and I hope you are looking down, proud of your little girl!

> *"The righteous man leads a blameless life; Blessed are his children after him."*
>
> —PROVERBS 20 7 NIV

ENTRY: 06/22 /20 (PART 1)

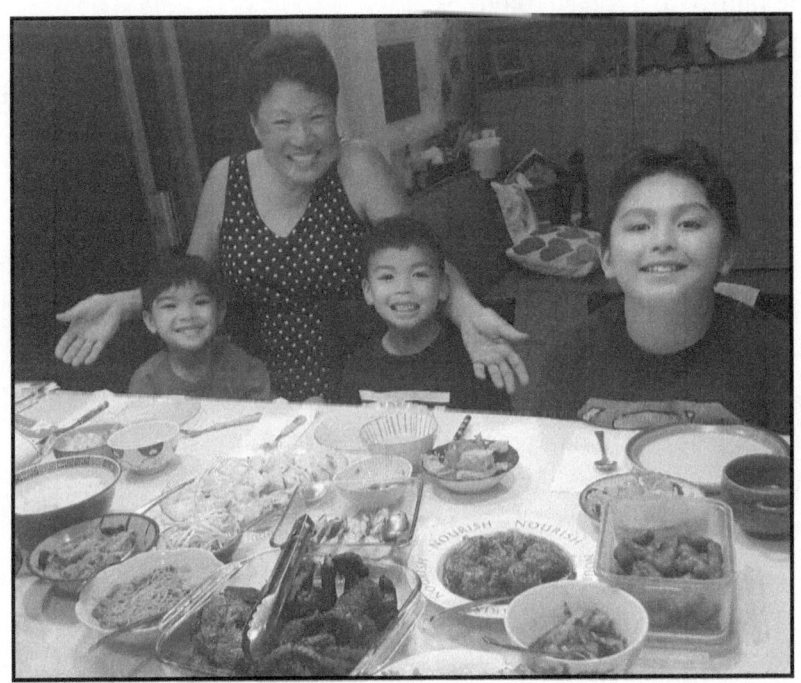

This COVID-19 pandemic has thrown so many of us off track. In the office, many of my family members and patients have been telling me that they have been eating more, staying up very late, and spending more time in front of screens than ever. Rapid weight gain has been typical, and everyone tells me they need to readjust and get healthier again. Parents have been telling me that it has been tough to maintain routines and regular meal schedules. However, this trend of being overweight or obese has been going on long before this pandemic started.

Over the years, as a pediatrician, I have been witnessing the rising trend of obesity in all ages, including parents. Currently, in addition to the COVID-19 pandemic, several factors contribute to this trend, including increased screen time, the loss of P.E. in schools, the rapid growth of fast-food chains, both parents working multiple jobs, less time for healthier home-cooked meals, and more. So, dear readers, over the following blogs, I'll share practical and basic information for everyone in the family to get back on track.

If I were even to start making a slight difference in this terrible trend, my mission would be to educate and include my young parents in healthy habits that would benefit not only their children but also their well-being. I always start by reminding parents that they are the "co-captains" or leaders of their family team. When their child is about six to nine months, I like to include them at the dinner table. When the family sits down for a meal, magical things begin to happen, and suddenly everyone is engaged in conversation.

Over the years, family meals have been extensively studied and repeatedly shown to have numerous benefits. For starters, family meals tend to be more nutritious and encourage everyone to eat a larger amount and variety of fruits and vegetables. People also tend to eat less during family meals because they eat more slowly and engage in more conversation. Additionally, family meals strengthen ties, build better relationships within the family, and give everyone a sense of belonging. Most important of all, the research shows that children who regularly eat family meals have a much lower chance of engaging in high-risk behaviors such as substance abuse, violence, and psychological problems.

The first and foremost thing for all of us to do is first recognize that there is a problem. Then, sit down as a family and discuss ways to tackle this problem.

One way to get started is for the entire family to get involved with meal planning, grocery shopping, food preparation, and even help with cooking, if they are old enough. The kids will feel great about helping and more likely eating their meals. Teach the children how to set the table and discuss proper table manners. Turn off the TVs, iPads, and phones, and let the family meal conversations begin.

In Okinawa, where people live extraordinarily long and healthy lives, there is a cultural practice they adhere to called "hara hachi bu." This practice is a constant reminder to stop eating when your stomach is 80 percent full. By simply practicing this culture of calorie restriction and mindful eating, the Okinawans have one of the highest percentages of centenarians anywhere else in the world.

The following tips can help you get started today:

- Eat more slowly. When you eat faster, you eat more.
- Focus on the food and keep the TVs, iPads, and phones of
- Choose to eat on smaller plates or bowls. By doing this, you can trick yourself into eating significantly less without even thinking about it.

So, practice being aware of how "full" you are feeling during your meal. If you are feeling stomach pressure, then you're probably getting 80 percent full. Another way to think about this is to eat until you are no longer hungry, rather than eating until you are full.

And once again, dear readers, because I cannot stress this enough: Let's make it a goal to have as many family meals as possible. Perhaps you, too, will see the many benefits of family meals unfold right before you.

> *"Do you not know that your bodies are temples of the Holy Spirit, who is in you, whom you have received from God?*
>
> *You are not your own; you were bought at a price. Therefore, honor God with your bodies."*
>
> —1 CORINTHIANS 6:19–20 NIV

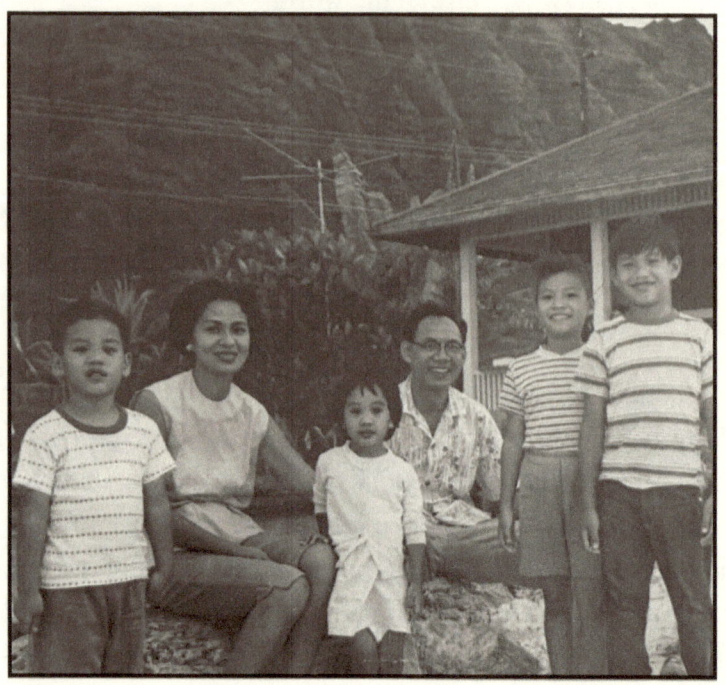

When growing up as a little girl, there were no twenty-four-hour fitness or UFC gyms. We had one black and white TV in our home, and there were only three channels to choose from, so screen time was boring. On the weekends or days off, my parents would make us play outside all day and only wanted us home by dinner time. We did not have many store-bought toys, but we used our imagination with boxes and anything else we could get our hands on.

My parents were constantly making a list of chores for us to do. They would always remind us that chores were good exercise for us, so they were doing this for our good. We had no dishwashers, and even though we had a clothes dryer, Mom rarely used it, so we had to hang the clothes outside. We never got allowances for doing chores, but we knew it was expected of us to help the family and contribute what we could.

Today's world is so different, and many children are no longer expected to do chores. Many parents hire a housekeeper to come in regularly, or they do it all themselves. When teens come home after school, they are not allowed outdoors and thus have unlimited screen time and a "free for all" of snacking at home. Sound familiar? During the COVID-19 quarantine, I believe that this stay-at-home order has exacerbated the problem. We are now living in the "perfect storm" for rapid weight gain to sneak its ugly head into our homes.

My solution for families is simple. Parents need to take back control of the situation. They need to make goals, schedules, and routines that everyone can agree upon and follow through. If grandparents live in the home, they too must be all in and help to enforce these rules. Finally, children should have their input taken under advisement but should never have equal voting rights as parents. Involving kids in major decisions that affect them makes compliance easier.

Remember, always remain flexible and adjust schedules or rules if they are not working. The next step should be to divide and delegate chores based on age and abilities, and these assignments should be enforced regularly.

The way I look at it, the sooner families can complete the essential chores, the more "free family time" they will have. Some of our best memories were the spontaneous family excursions we took with our four children, such as hikes, bike rides, or just having a picnic lunch outdoors.

I learned very quickly that our children don't need more things, but instead, they want a regular, predictable time together with us. If we can make family time a priority, whether it's during meals, chores, or just enjoying free time together, I promise that connectedness, respect, and happiness are bound to follow.

At this time in our country, I believe it is more critical than ever to get things straight within the family first. If our families succeed, our nation also succeeds.

"How good and pleasant it is when God's people live together in unity."

—PSALM 133:1 NIV

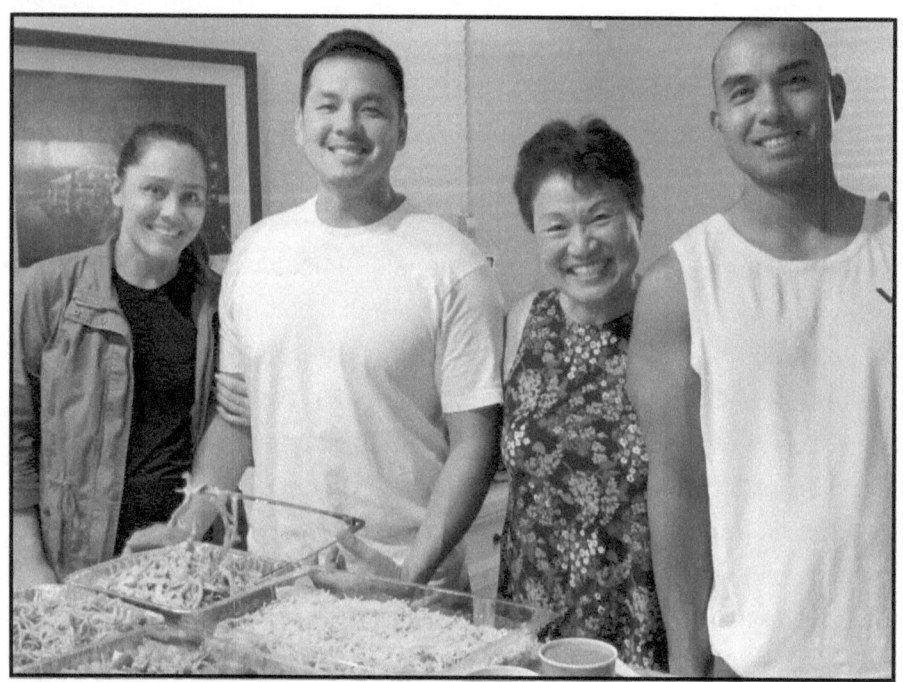

Our news media continues to inundate us with conflicting advice about ways to "avoid" getting or spreading COVID-19. Today, I wanted to share another vital way to fight this virus. The key is to strengthen your immune system from within your body. Several factors contribute to maintaining our immune system at full capacity, including adequate sleep, regular exercise, stress relief or mindfulness, and the foods we eat daily.

Just as this pandemic has put the spotlight on handwashing, I wanted to focus on the types of foods that help strengthen our immune system today. In other words, ask yourself: How will this food impact me? Currently, the standard American diet consists of many foods that cause our bodies to be "chronically inflamed."

Let me explain. Your immune system is your home security system, and "inflammation" is the alarm. In our bodies' case, the invader can be a virus, a bruised hand, or an allergic reaction to pollen. In a well-functioning immune system, it will eventually disarm.

Research now shows that a significant contributor to "chronic inflammation" is the foods we eat daily. Some major culprits include sugar (in sodas and candy), processed foods, vegetable oils, fried foods, refined flour, artificial sweeteners and additives, saturated fats, and a second round of alcohol. As a result, our immune system alarm is never disarmed, and this will then lead to many problems such as infections, weight gain, cancer, digestive issues, fatigue, diabetes, and more.

Food tastes and choices are so ingrained in us that, for the most part, we are not mindful about what we eat daily. Convenience, taste, and costs frequently make healthier food choices very difficult. However, if everyone understands the importance of eating more nutritious foods and fewer junk foods, then compliance becomes easier.

So, dear readers, let's not obsess over the latest quick-fix fad diet or pill that will make you healthier and lose weight instantly. Instead, let's focus on daily foods that benefit us, especially those that boost our immune system. Some examples of these beneficial or "non-inflammatory" foods include fatty fish, berries, avocados, green tea, peppers, mushrooms, cherries, tomatoes, extra-virgin olive oil, and dark chocolate.

I always share with my patients the "Try a bite rule." Everyone in the family, including adults, is encouraged to try a new fruit or vegetable a few bites at a time. Studies show that after seven to ten tries, most people will start to like this new food.

As we all know, any permanent change takes time. The slower the change, the more permanent the change. It is crucial that the entire family stay focused and encouraged. Another rule I share is that there's no such thing as "forbidden foods." Everything in moderation. So, if you have been diligent with your food choices the entire week, reward yourselves on the weekend with an evening out for dinner or an ice cream treat.

Remember, significant changes often begin with parents or grandparents making informed choices about the food they buy and preparing tasty, healthy meals at home. By making even the most minor changes daily, you and your family will soon reap the rewards of an improved immune system, more energy, fewer illnesses, and perhaps, even some weight loss for adults.

> *"I appeal to you therefore, brothers, by the mercies of God, to present your bodies as a living sacrifice, holy and acceptable to God, which is your spiritual worship."*
>
> —ROMANS 12:1 NIV

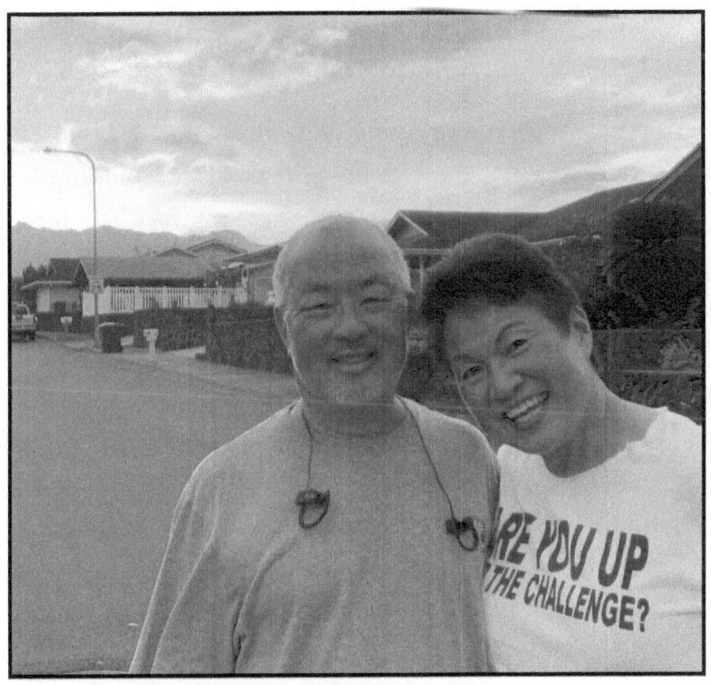

During this COVID-19 pandemic, I wanted to share with you my experience as a patient today. I had my follow-up colonoscopy, and as a physician, I thought it was a good exercise to write about what it felt like to be on "the other side" as a patient.

No one likes undergoing a colonoscopy, but I understand the necessity of this procedure. For those who have never had one, it's thirty-six hours of prep before the procedure to clean out your bowels, which's the worst. To get the best results, your entire digestive tract needs to be pristinely cleaned out. Thus, twenty-four hours before the procedure, it's a liquid diet that also includes drinking a gallon of nasty-tasting fluid. On the way over, Martin held my hand, said a prayer over me, and I felt much better.

In this "new normal" of COVID-19, anyone undergoing a procedure at the hospital must now undergo COVID-19 testing two days prior. I'm happy to report that I had a negative COVID-19 result, but I must confess the swab used to get the specimen in the back of your nose was uncomfortable for those ten seconds.

When I registered early this morning at the hospital, it felt sterile with signs everywhere reminding you that we are still deep in this COVID-19 pandemic. The registrar wore her face mask and sat behind the plastic "spit guard." She put on gloves before picking up my ID and insurance card, and then had me sanitize my hands before I picked up the pen to sign my name. As I sat in the sparsely furnished, empty waiting room, with chairs spaced six to ten feet apart, I felt a deep sense of loneliness.

I was finally called back to the area to prepare for my procedure. As I removed all my clothes and put on the hospital gown, which opens in the back, I suddenly felt very vulnerable… the first thought that came to me was that I hoped my doctor got a good night's sleep for his job today. I wonder if any of my patients ever asks that question about me?

Several nurses came to help me, all wearing face masks, face shields, and constantly sanitizing their hands. It's strange not to see people's entire faces, but I'm learning to look into their eyes to see the caring spirit in them. I know these health care workers do this same drill day in and day out, but they made me feel very comfortable and put me at ease. They kept telling me everything they were doing and what to expect next. Funny how just a little grateful smile under my mask made them smile back at me, even though I couldn't see their faces.

They finally rolled me into the procedure room, and there was the familiar, smiling face of my doctor. He looked well rested and came to my bedside to talk to me. The last words I heard from him were, "Don't worry, everything will be fine. I need to keep you around for many more years." I smiled, got my fentanyl sedative, and took a good nap.

The entire hospital visit lasted four hours, and I was pleased with the experience, despite my initial apprehensions. My wonderful husband, Martin, was on standby and drove me home. I had a small lunch, a great nap, and sat down to write today's blog.

Dear readers, if you are overdue for a colonoscopy or any other necessary procedure at the hospital, please do not postpone it. Please know that it's not as bad as you think, and it could potentially save your life.

> *" 'But I will restore you to health and heal your wounds,' declares the Lord, 'because you are called an outcast, Zion for whom no one cares.' "*

—JEREMIAH 30:17 NIV

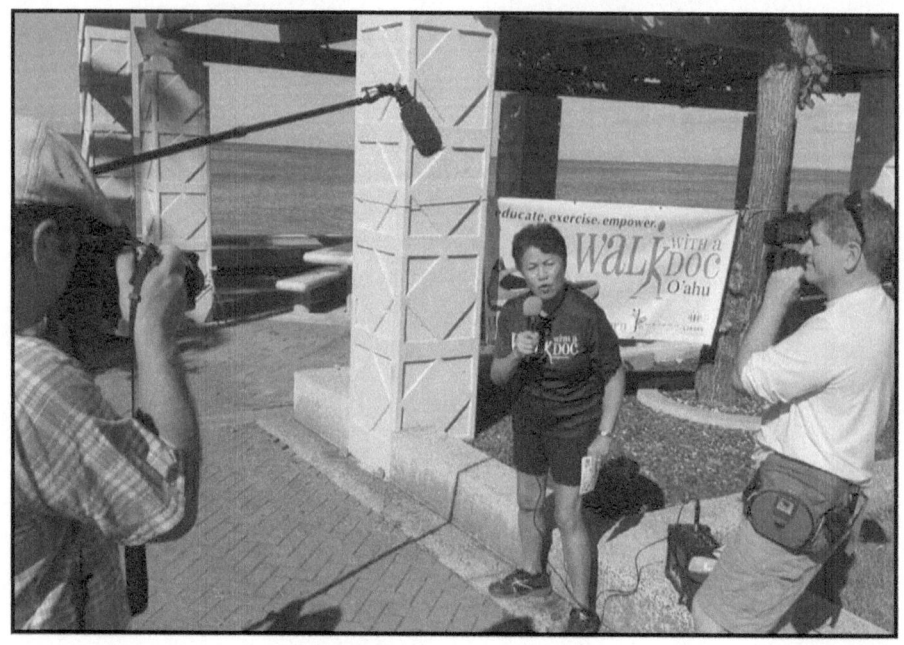

appy Aloha Friday, everyone! I'm feeling much better after my procedure yesterday. My husband has been treating me like a queen, and we've been spending a lot of quality time together as I recuperate from my procedure. He told me he enjoys hearing my insights, as a physician, on various topics. I wanted to share some thoughts I have on being a physician and what it means to be a "primary care physician."

First, I feel that physicians have a reputation of being "gods" and knowing all the answers to any medical question. Well, I'll let you in on a secret… we don't always know everything. Yes, we've all undergone rigorous training and education after completing four years of medical school, followed by three to five years of specialty residency training. However, we are also constantly learning new information and gaining more experience with each passing year. I would also like to add that we certainly have more education, training, and credibility than people who post "medical information" on social media.

Over the past thirty-five years of practice, the way we treat patients has undergone drastic changes. Instead of just ordering our patients to do the list of things we tell them, we are now finding better outcomes when we work as a team and collaborate with our patients and families. In other words, physicians and their staff work together with patients to achieve the best possible medical outcome and experience, as well as improved costs.

As I work with my patients and families, I attempt to individualize their care. In other words, one size does not always fit all. For example, when discussing weight and BMI (body mass index), if it falls into the overweight or obese category, I first ask my patient if they are ready for change. If they are, we move on to discuss what their priority for change is and how I can assist them in achieving it. By communicating effectively with each other, we can identify one or two initial changes to implement and then follow up, either in person or via telehealth, to keep everyone motivated.

The key point here is that your primary care physician serves as your "medical home," where ongoing chronic problems and concerns can be effectively addressed. The problem with only visiting Urgent Care Clinics or the ER is that the new physician you see on each visit has no knowledge of your medical history and may not fully understand the scope of your problems. If possible, I always urge my patients to call me or come in for care whenever it is possible.

Another rather obvious point to remember is that your physician is not a mind reader. It is okay to stop me and ask questions, tell me to slow down, or ask me to use simpler medical terminology. However, if you nod your head "yes" and seem to indicate that you understand everything, then that is what I'll believe.

Regarding appointment times, during the COVID-19 pandemic, please keep your appointments and arrive on time, as many patients are being turned away, and your spot in the schedule is extremely valuable. So, dear readers, please remember to stay in touch with your primary care physician, especially during this pandemic, as this is crucial for receiving the best possible medical care. It is now safe to visit your physician in the office, and telehealth virtual visits are also an option.

> *"Let your conversations be always full of grace, seasoned with salt, so that you may know how to answer everyone."*
>
> —COLOSSIANS 4:6 NIV

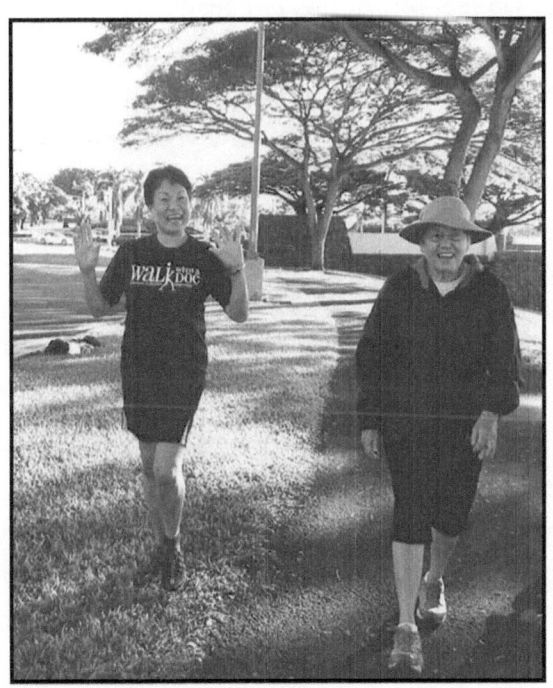

As I mentioned earlier, many of us have been quarantined at home, and the pandemic pounds have slowly crept in. It's time to decide to get back into the exercise routine, but how can we motivate ourselves to take that first step? Today, I wanted to share with you a valuable rule to help you transition from an idea to acting. This is called the "five-second rule." And I don't mean the five-second, where a piece of fallen food may be eaten if it was on the ground for less than five seconds.

This rule was first introduced in a famous TED Talk podcast by Mel Robbins and has since become one of the most-watched podcasts in the world.

Mel Robbins states that "knowing will never be enough." It is never as easy as the Nike slogan says to "Just do it." If it were all that simple, everyone would have everything they ever wanted.

Here is the problem. When we are confronted with what we should do versus what we feel like doing, our feelings will always prevail.

Within five seconds, your brain will come up with every excuse or hopeless thought on why you should not do this. This is called the "spotlighting effect," and that's just how your brain is wired to protect you from danger.

For example, if you make a decision you have been meaning to do for a while, such as calling your son and touching base, you could apply this five-second rule as follows: The weekend arrives and so immediately, you grab the five-second rule, start counting backwards as you dial, and focus on your commitment to chat with him. Voila! You speak with him and the family and feel so proud of finally taking that first step to move into action.

This is a proven strategy to do the hard stuff: the work you don't feel like doing or fear. Thousands of lives have been transformed for the better, just by practicing this. For myself, I learned about the five-second rule about four years ago and have been practicing it in my own life with much success. I wish I had been aware of this rule earlier.

The take-home message today is to start practicing the five-second rule in everyday life. Remember, practice makes perfect. When Saturday arrives, set your alarm for 7:00 a.m., count backward out loud (five, four, three, two, one, go), and get yourself moving. See you at the park!

"I have fought the good fight, I have finished the race, I have kept the faith."

—2 TIMOTHY 4 7 NIV

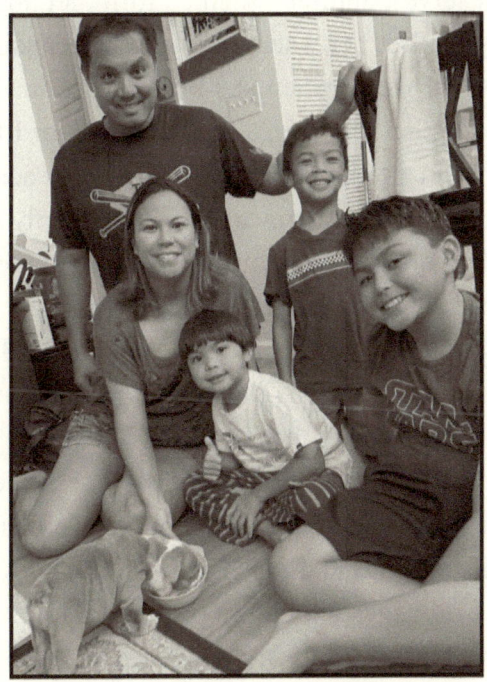

recently read an article about how dog adoptions and sales soared during the COVID-19 pandemic. I believe many people were trying to fill the void with their dogs or puppies. People everywhere were suddenly stuck at home with children who needed something to do, adults with no work, and lots of free time, or people simply feeling lonely with no way to socialize.

During the COVID-19 pandemic, my three active grandsons have been socially "safer at home," but they feel very restless and often bored. They are ten, six, and four years old and highly active. Due to the pandemic, they have been spending a considerable amount of time on their iPads. When the opportunity came up for my son and daughter-in-law to get the puppy of her dreams, she jumped at the chance.

The other night, we were invited to visit Pebbles Wee, the new addition to their family. The cutest observation of the night was seeing our three grandsons interact with her and focusing their attention on her every move. I thought it was great for the boys to think of someone else besides themselves, and they seemed to forget about their screens completely. They fetched her water, threw away her soiled pee pad, and even ran to get toilet tissue when she began to poop. They spent time cuddling and kissing her tenderly, a type of behavior I have rarely seen from these boys. I can already see that this dog will teach them kindness, responsibility, and love. I'm happy to see that not only are their screens turned off, but they are very anxious to go outdoors to walk, run, and play with her, once she gets her vaccines.

As boys, this new pet is now offering them an excellent opportunity to develop their nurturing skills. I think the boys feel safe taking care of their dog and feel it's not like they're doing a "girl" thing, like playing house or with dolls. Additionally, when everyone shares in the care of the family pet, it fosters an additional bond, as well as increased communication among siblings and parents.

I think our world needs a lot more of this right now. In our COVID pandemic and our nation's unrest, we need parents to do their best to teach their children good values of respect and responsibility.

> *"Let everything that has breath praise the Lord. Praise the Lord."*
>
> —PSALM 150:6 NIV

5

JULY

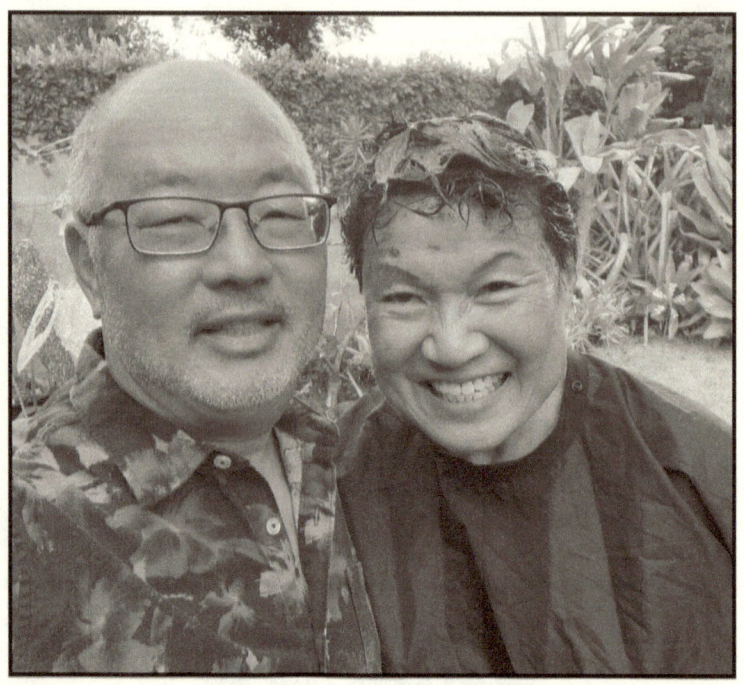

don't know about you, dear readers, but, frankly, I'm getting a bit exhausted and fed up with this virus. I read an article yesterday in my medical journal talking about "quarantine fatigue." Yes, this is a genuine medical diagnosis, and it resonated with me. For months on end now, we've all had to make sacrifices, isolate at home, and have had to get used to the loss of freedom to go about life as we did "pre-quarantine."

I often feel like stress and anxiety keep piling up, and there sometimes seems to be no relief in sight. Due to the protracted nature of the COVID-19 pandemic, along with the daily news of unrest in our nation and around the world, it feels like it all contributes to a pervasive sense of fatigue.

I thought of an analogy that might help you relate to this feeling. Think of your cell phone that has a limited amount of energy before it needs recharging. Humans are very similar in that we can only function for so long before we become depleted, slow down, and eventually shut off if we don't get recharged.

After a three-hour conference last night, I was physically and emotionally exhausted, tired, hungry, and ready to drive home. I called Martin to let him know I was on my way home, and to my surprise, he was waiting for me at the nearby Pacific Club with dinner reservations. We had a wonderful, satisfying, and delicious dinner with lots of great conversation. It was great to be out on a date with my husband.

Before going to bed last night, I thought about the fantastic conclusion to my day. It made me feel happy to focus on the blessings in my life, despite all the negative "stuff" going on around me. I know I've said this before, but we all need to remember to pause and focus on the good stuff that happens all around us, day in and day out. It's so easy to fall into that dark black hole of negativity.

Some examples of my blessings yesterday included a great pep talk from my office manager; a grateful mother reminding me that twenty-five years ago, I was her pediatrician; a hard-working staff that got me out on time a bit earlier yesterday; my gastroenterologist calling me to tell me that my two polyps were benign and that I had one of the cleanest and healthiest looking colons… and most of all, a loving husband who goes out of his way to care for me, treats me like a queen, and makes me laugh often.

He even trimmed and colored my hair this past weekend again with a cheerful heart. He has great precision and thoroughness in his work, and I appreciated him spending several hours of his weekend doing this for me. Now that is true love!

Yes, dear readers, I may have "quarantine fatigue," but I am counteracting it with the many blessings in my life. The key takeaway from today's blog is to pause every evening and be grateful for the many blessings that come our way each day.

"Rejoice always, pray continually, give thanks in all circumstances; for this is God's will for you in Christ Jesus."

—1 THESSALONIANS 5:16–18 NIV

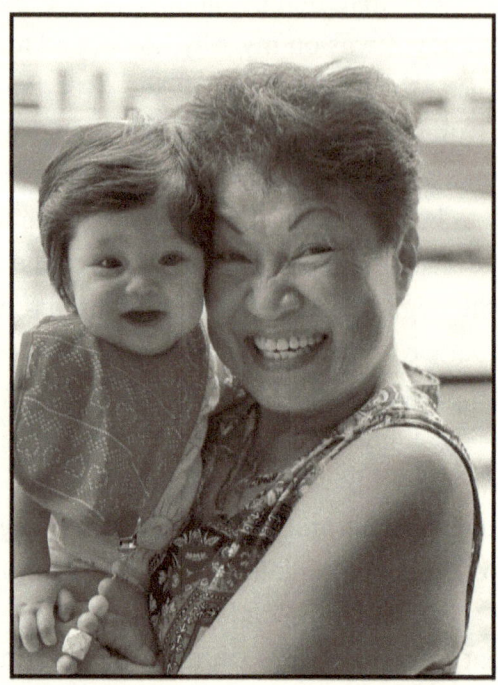

I have breaking news to share with all of you today: My beautiful granddaughter, Karter Ellie Wee, was born early this morning. Both mother and daughter are doing well. I have been praying for this day to arrive, as I have been very concerned about the possibility of Samantha getting COVID-19 during her pregnancy.

My son sent me a text last night saying that Samantha was admitted to the hospital, and I kept getting up every two hours, checking my phone for any news. As a pediatrician for many years, I have seen a great deal, and although everything goes well 99.99 percent of the time, a constant little voice in my head is always on guard for all possibilities. I'm happy to report that at 5:40 AM, I finally got the text stating that she arrived safely and is a healthy baby girl!

It was great to see my son, Chris, step up to the plate and be such a caring, responsible, and protective husband. He took all the necessary precautions. As a mother, there is nothing more satisfying than seeing your children become the adults you always imagined they could be.

I also want to give kudos to my daughter-in-law, Samantha, who took great care of herself throughout this pandemic. There was always the possibility of COVID-19 infection looming, but she did social isolation and all other measures to stay healthy.

Finally, there is Khloe, Karter's ten-year-old sister, who is thrilled to have a new sister. She has been excited about her baby sister from the beginning and can't wait to be a big helper for Mom and Dad.

Karter is our fifth grandchild (sixth if you count our new addition, Pebbles, the English Lilac Bulldog), and Martin and I are ecstatic.

As I continue to stare at this photo of Karter, I am filled with great hope for the future. She is a precious gift and blessing from the Lord, and I know she will be in good hands with these parents.

Every child is precious in God's eyes and deserves to be loved, nurtured, protected, and enabled to develop to their full potential. It takes a village to raise our children in a healthy, happy, loving, safe, caring environment where their needs are met. So, the take-home message today is whenever you see opportunities to advocate, improve, help, or show love to a child, please act. Our children depend on us even more during these uncertain times.

So, congratulations, Chris and Samantha! We're so happy for you and can't wait to meet Miss Karter Wee!

"The word of the Lord came to me, saying, 'Before I formed you in the womb, I knew you; before you were born, I set you apart; I appointed you as a prophet to the nations.'"

—JEREMIAH 1:4–5 NIV

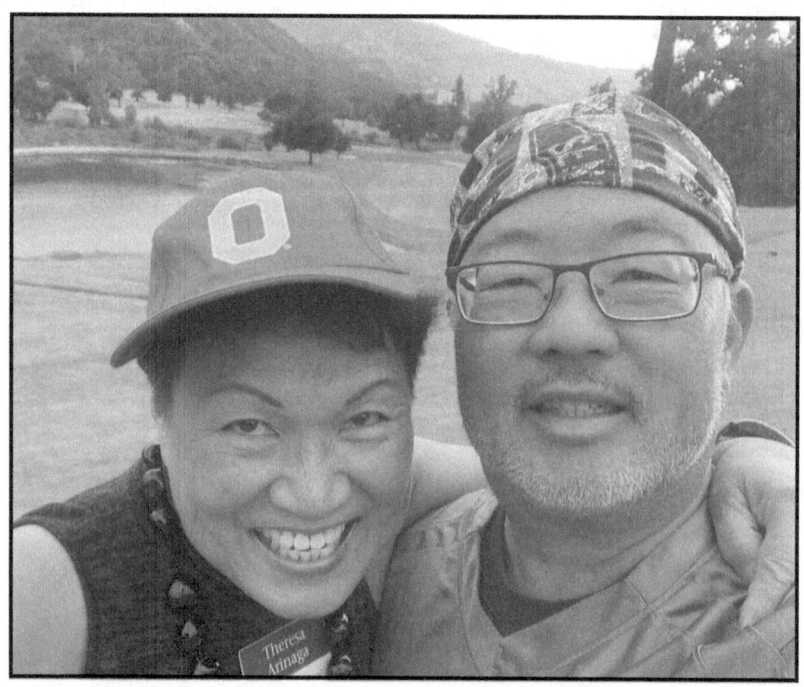

On this eve of July 4, 2020, I cannot help but think of our great nation. Even though we cannot have our traditional gatherings to watch the fireworks and other annual celebrations, it is still important to pause and reflect on our great nation. I listened to a radio show today, and it made numerous references to one of our greatest U.S. presidents, Ronald Reagan. As a result, I spent most of today listening to many of his memorable speeches on YouTube. I thought it would be appropriate to share some ideas and new insights that I learned from this great American.

Every day on our televisions, social media, and newspapers, we read about the mayhem, discontent, and violence going on in nearly all our major cities. Some people now want to get rid of the Fourth of July holiday, defund our police force, and ridicule anyone who loves our country.

As an "older "American, I recall being raised very differently from the youth of today. At home, I was taught to love our great country and remember my parents' efforts in helping relatives immigrate to America in search of a better life. Patriotism seemed to be everywhere in our neighborhoods, and nearly all the dads I knew growing up had served in the military. At school, we said the Pledge of Allegiance every morning, with our right hand over our heart. Even the television shows and movies we watched celebrated the great values of America, reminding us of how exceptional our nation was.

Sadly, times have changed. I feel that our younger generation is not getting the message of why our country is so great. True American history is no longer being taught in some schools, and children are not receiving the complete story of our founding fathers' efforts to form a unique government experiment, never attempted before anywhere else in the world.

President Reagan stated in his memorable farewell speech that our great nation still stands steady after more than 200 years, despite the storms she had had to endure. I am confident that we will get through this as well. America is a shining beacon of hope for freedom to the world, and we must bring her back to her full glory. Our founders said we were one nation under God, and God intended for us to be free.

So, dear readers, today's blog serves as a reminder to each of us to have the courage to be part of the "resurgence of patriotism" or "the New Patriotism Revolution," a term coined by President Reagan that is even more relevant at this time. In other words, as American citizens, we must each put forth our best effort to believe that together, and with God's help, we can resolve any problem that confronts us. But this will take effort by each one of us to teach our youth the truth of America's history, stand up for what is right, and make the necessary sacrifices to protect our great nation and valuable freedom for future generations.

President Reagan said that there is no greater weapon in the world than the will and moral courage of free people. It is a message to our enemies of freedom that we will never surrender our freedom, and we will hold peace as our highest aspiration, for we are Americans.

As I close this blog tonight, I wish you all God's blessings, dear readers, and God bless America. Happy Birthday, America! I am so proud to be an American citizen!

> *"You, my brothers, were called to be free. But do not use your freedom to indulge in the sinful nature; rather, serve one another in love. For the entire law is summed up in a single command: 'Love your neighbor as yourself."*

> —GALATIANS:5:13–14 NIV

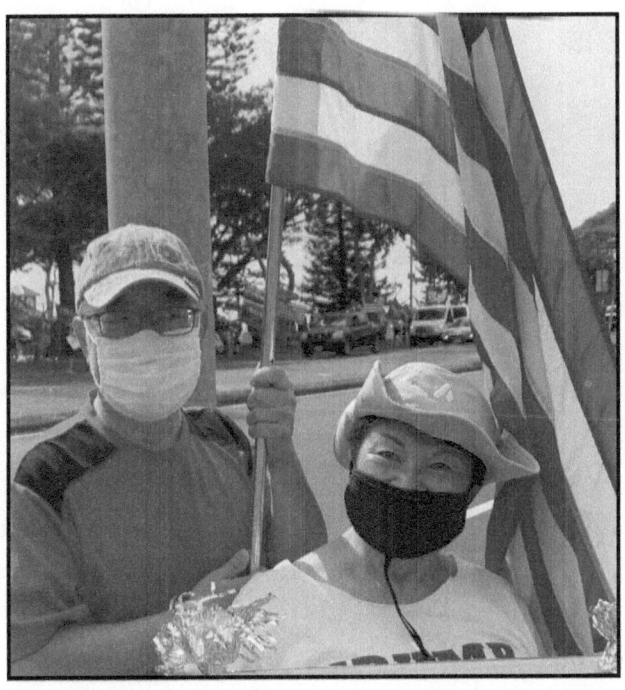

H appy July 4, dear readers! To celebrate this special holiday, Martin and I took the day to drive around the island. It has been years since we did this, and we just wanted to have a change of scenery. It was so much fun!

I love having "windshield time" with my husband and we always have good conversations about many topics, including COVID-19, as well as the current affairs of our state and country. Currently, I'm deeply saddened by the terrible events unfolding across our nation. I consider myself part of the "silent majority" and I just can't take this anymore.

As an American patriot, my heart is deeply saddened at the violence, tearing down of historical monuments and memorials, vandalism of private property, destruction of businesses, and much more. Today, I need to voice my opinion. The people doing these horrible things want us to be scared and fearful of them; they think we are weak and won't speak up. But they are wrong. I am not going to allow them to attack my freedom, and I will do everything to protect my family, business, and liberty.

In 1776, the Declaration of Independence was written, stating that we believe our rights are "inalienable," which means they cannot be given or taken away. If we live by this, then we see everyone as worthy of love and respect. We do not have these rights because we earned them or because of the color of our skin or gender. We have these rights because God deemed that we were made in his image and likeness.

Christianity shaped our nation, and our foundation was built on Biblical ideas. As Christianity declines, we see more people in our country looking more favorably on the idea of more government involvement. Instead of turning to God, they want the government to solve their problems. A perfect example of this is in China. The Chinese Communist Party continues to place restrictions on religious freedom, is not accountable to voters, censors all internet use, and much more. As the government gains power, the people lose power.

What our nation needs now are people who look to God once again and reflect Christ in all that we do. Our foundation as a Christian nation needs people who are willing to fight for these very ideas.

So, dear readers, stop being part of the "silent majority." We all need to speak out and fight for our country.

> "But seek first his kingdom and his righteousness, and all these things will be given to you as well."
>
> —MATTHEW 6:33 NIV

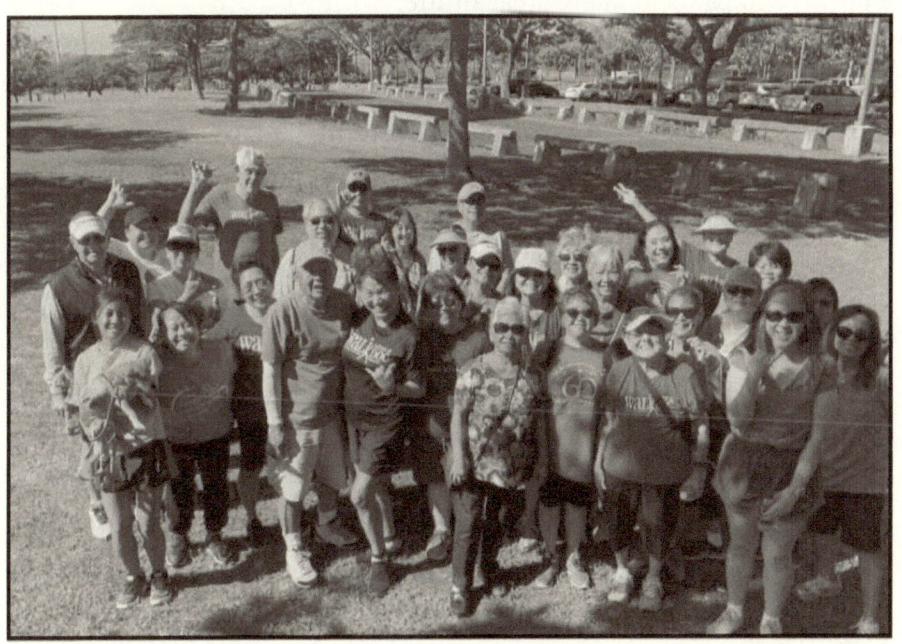

Today, I wanted to discuss the topic of self-control. I thought I would bring up this topic because many families have been telling me how difficult it has been during the COVID-19 pandemic to eat healthily and stay disciplined with an exercise regimen.

One definition of self-control is the ability to resist short-term temptation and instead follow through with plans that are beneficial for the future.

So, let's dive in and see what's so great about learning self-control? A well-known marshmallow test was conducted on four-year-old children in the 1960s. These children were told that if they didn't eat the marshmallow for fifteen minutes, then they would receive a second one and could have both marshmallows. Well, after fifteen minutes, two out of three children went ahead and ate the marshmallow. Years later, it was found that those who were able to delay gratification to receive a greater reward were less likely to be overweight, use fewer drugs, and had higher SAT scores. The conclusion was that self-control tends have a positive impacts in many areas of life.

We all have seen self-control go out the window when it comes to our health. A recent survey by the American Psychological Association found that 27 percent of respondents identified a lack of willpower as the primary factor keeping them from reaching their goals. However, don't despair; researchers say there are several factors and strategies to improve your self-control.

If you are working towards a goal, then three things must be present:

- A clear goal and the motivation to change. An example might be to walk three times a week to get back on track toward better health.
- Track your progress toward achieving the goal. Simply setting a goal isn't enough. Monitor and record your behavior to ensure you're doing the necessary things to reach your goal. Finally, you have the willpower or self-control to modify your behavior.

Here are some tips for improving self-control:

1. Avoid temptation – For example, when we are quarantined at home and have too many tempting desserts in our kitchen, it's so easy to give in. Studies show that we have a fixed amount of energy to resist temptation, and once it's gone, we give in. The common-sense solution, of course, would be not to have these types of food in your home to begin with.
2. Plan – Consider possible situations that might break your resolve. Research shows that planning can improve willpower.
3. Practice using self-control – Think of self-control as a muscle. Over time, as you repeatedly use this muscle, it will grow stronger.
4. Focus on one goal at a time – It is always best to choose only one specific goal at the beginning and focus all your energy on this.

5. Mindfulness meditation – This is a great way to learn to slow your thoughts and help control your impulses getting in the way of your self-control.
6. Remind yourself of the consequences.

As we slowly emerge from the social isolation caused by the pandemic, let us all consider setting a specific goal to improve our health and exercise self-control to achieve it.

> *"The plans of the diligent lead to profit as surely as haste leads to poverty."*
>
> —PROVERBS 21:5 NIV

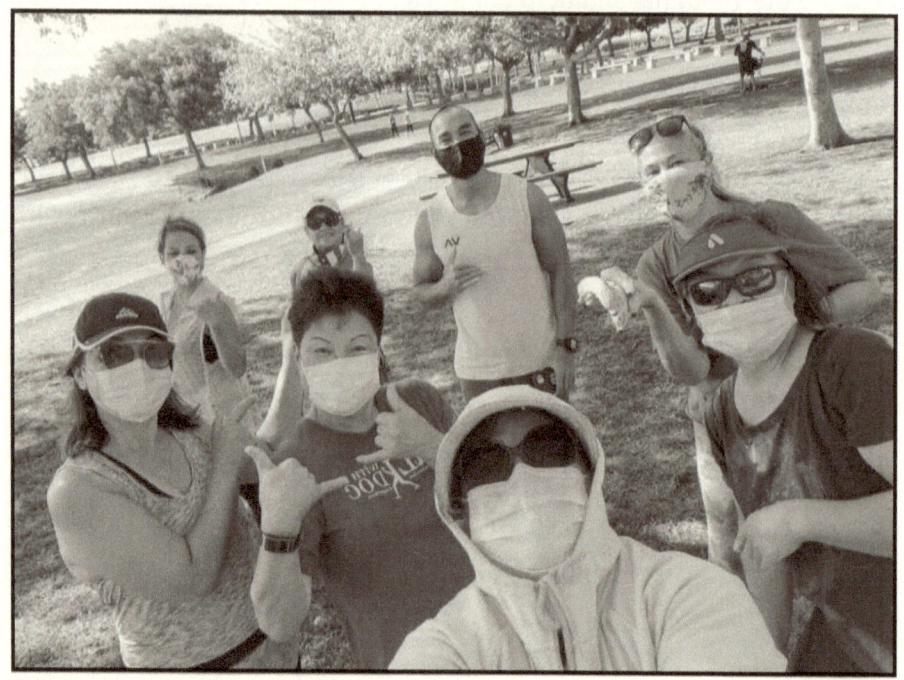

In this COVID-19 pandemic, I continue seeing families with lots of challenges due to social isolation with their children as well as parents having no choice but to be at home due to layoffs or being forced to work from home. This is an unprecedented and challenging time, and being a parent during the pandemic is no picnic. It is just plain hard work, and problematic situations arise daily. This is the time when we, as parents, must muster up the grit and perseverance to endure these storms. It also helps to keep a sense of humor and know that you are not alone in this.

My husband, Stephen, got very creative and found innovative ways to get our kids to cooperate. He rarely needed to raise his voice and creatively devised humorous strategies to teach them lessons they would remember for the rest of their lives.

Our three boys would constantly fight with each other, and for the most part, we allowed them to work things out on their own. Stephen's famous reminder was always "just don't get blood on the carpet and watch out for those expensive braces." Another time, when the kids refused to come out to say goodbye to Grandma and Grandpa, he would have the kids stand out there waving goodbye until their hands were so sore that they couldn't raise them anymore. The next time the grandparents left, they all came running out to wave goodbye.

One of the most important lessons I learned as a parent was always to let them know that I believed in them. We needed to stick with them through thick and thin, but ultimately, it was up to them to make the choices, good or bad, and then learn from them.

I always believe that we, as parents, are constantly striving to do the best we can to provide the most stable and nurturing environment for them. However, despite our good intentions, there are many things that we get wrong, and parenting often seems like a trial-and-error process. What we need to remember is that we are not the only parents out there struggling with challenges… so hold onto the small glimmer of hope that tomorrow will be a better day. God only wants us to love our children and do our best… that's all we can do. We may not see the rewards of our labor for decades, but God desires for us to be faithful and patient, one day at a time.

The take-home message for all parents is to get back up each time after being knocked down. Embrace the support of family, friends, and the community to help and persevere day after day… our children are depending on us.

> *"Trust in the Lord with all your heart and lean not on your own understanding; in all your ways submit to him, and he will make your paths straight. Do not be wise in your own eyes; fear the Lord and shun evil. This will bring health to your body and nourishment to your bones."*
>
> —PROVERBS 3:5–8 NIV

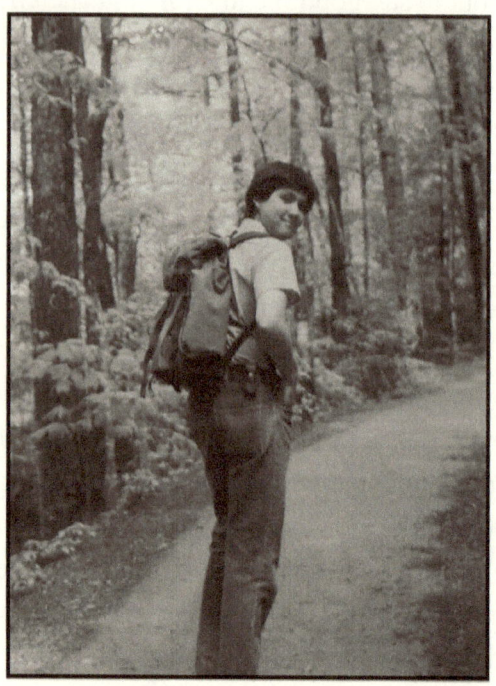

Recently, I've been thinking a lot about parenting, perhaps because I'm a new "Grammy" once again. As a pediatrician, I'm constantly addressing parenting issues with my families, as it is so essential for them to be the leaders in their family. I feel it is easier to prepare our children at an early age for life, rather than try to repair them as adults.

As parents, we go through day-to-day events such as meals, bath time, homework, and laundry, among others. It is a daily grind, and each day seems like an eternity. I remember one day, I felt so overwhelmed, I looked at my four young children and asked them, "When are you all going to grow up?" Well, I didn't get an answer, only surprised looks.

People always tell me that before you know it, your children will all be grown up. I never believed them, until it happened to me! They were correct. At each of their high school or college graduations, I always wondered if my husband and I had spent enough time with them.

As I mentioned before, Stephen and I spent six days a week seeing patients in our private medical practices. Time with the family was limited, but I want to share some ways we made the most of it. Weekends were precious and the best time to do family activities. Stephen and I planned lunch picnics, beach outings, hikes, bike riding as a family, fishing excursions, walking around the airport, or just about anything we could do together. It didn't have to be an expensive outing... if we were together, that was all that mattered.

At home, Stephen was so good about including the kids in his "man cave," his well-organized garage workshop. This was also the gathering place for the neighborhood men, as well as the meetings of the Cub Scouts and Boy Scouts. As soon as the sound of the electric saw came on, everyone would come over to see what the next project was. Stephen made bed frames, drawers, a tree house, a "lemonade stand," a skateboard ramp, and set decorations for recitals, among other things, with everyone pitching in to help. To this day, all four of my children continue to amaze me with their carpentry skills as well as renovations on their homes. I now realize that children need to observe their parents, caretakers, and teachers, as they quickly absorb more than they think.

One of the most important lessons my husband modeled on for me was the importance of being present in the moment with your children, or anyone, for that matter. It sounds simple, but it's not always easy when you have a hundred other things on your mind. Stephen was a pro at this, and anyone who encountered him could attest to this. You always felt special when speaking with him, knowing you had his undivided attention.

Time keeps ticking by, so we all need to make the most of it, especially with our loved ones. To have a meaningful and intimate relationship with loved ones, we must clear our minds and be fully present in those precious moments with them.

We often hear at lucky drawings, "You must be present to win." I would agree that this saying is true of life.

"Be very careful, then, how you live – not as unwise but as wise, making the most of every opportunity, because the days are evil. Therefore, do not be foolish, but understand what the Lord's will is."

—EPHESIANS 5:15–17 NIV

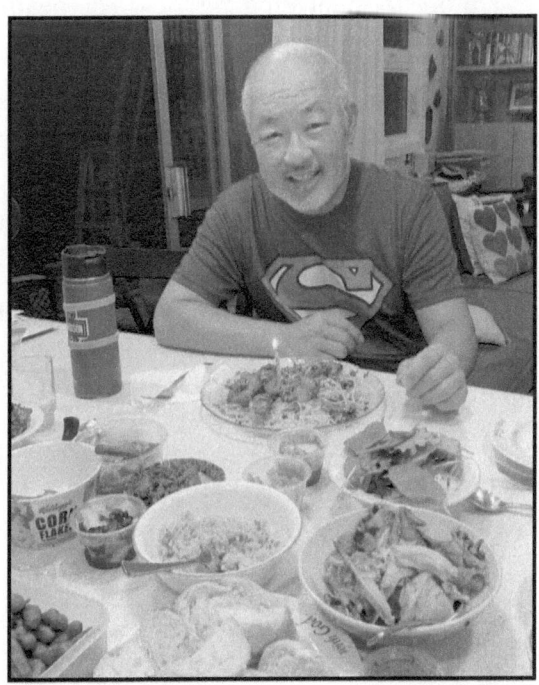

During these days of confinement, I'm often seeing people turning to their comfort foods to calm their anxieties. Sales have doubled and, in some cases, tripled for cookies, salty snacks like chips, and ice cream. Other categories of food that people are stocking up on include macaroni and cheese, rice, and chocolates. Even alcoholic beverage sales have also spiked during this pandemic.

Today, I wanted to talk about an alternative way of coping with our fears, anxiety, and uncertainties. I want to discuss "mindfulness." I know this term may be foreign to many of you, but the more I learn about this, the more I realize its numerous benefits.

Every morning, we wake up, God has given us another twenty-four hours to live and make a difference in this world. We have this gift of another day to bring joy and happiness to ourselves and others.

Let's start each day by practicing mindfulness by setting the intention to be fully present and in the moment. When we pay close attention to what we are doing, we experience more peace of mind and calmness as we work through our thoughts and worries. The healing benefits of mindfulness include acknowledging our feelings, such as anxiety and fearfulness, gaining insight into their underlying causes, and adopting a more courageous and inquisitive attitude toward our experiences.

As an exercise, I want each of you, right now, to sit upright with feet on the ground and take a full breath through your nose. Hold it for a moment, then fully exhale through your mouth till your breath is all out. Repeat this exercise three times and do it two or three times throughout the day. By doing this, you will remind yourself to be fully present with all your senses and feelings and then reset your intentions to be mindful in your daily activities.

A great time to practice being mindful is when we are eating our meals. Instead of just shoveling it into our mouths, take a moment to think about what we're choosing to eat, then look at the colors of the food, smell the different aromas, and feel the different textures as you chew the food in your mouth and taste each morsel you eat. Finally, throughout the meal, feel and express appreciation for the efforts that went into preparing this meal and the blessing of having an abundance of food. This combination of mindfulness and gratitude can connect us to this moment and bring us much joy, not to mention helping us eat less and healthier.

Remember, dear readers, think of mindfulness not as something to be done "as needed," like Tylenol for a headache, but rather like brushing your teeth regularly several times a day. Establish the intention to be as steady as possible in practicing to be fully present throughout your day.

As we prepare to sleep at night, take a few moments to reflect and be grateful for another day. Remember that God, our loving Father, is always an integral part of our daily lives. Jesus was a great example of being mindful. He was focused on His Heavenly Father and the Kingdom of God. He trusted that everything was in His Father's hands. As a result, he was always fully present to everyone he encountered.

"Test me, Lord, and try me, examine my heart and my mind; for I have always been mindful of your unfailing love and have lived in reliance on your faithfulness."

—PSALM 26:2–3 NIV

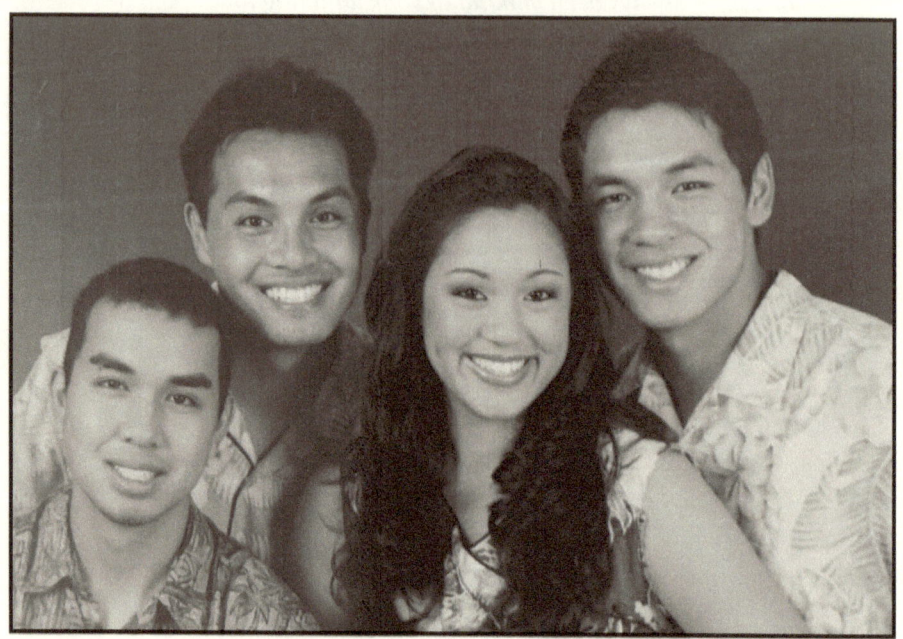

As this pandemic continues with no end in sight, parents share with me their struggles daily. Sometimes, it seems overwhelming, and you're never sure if you're doing the right thing.

Today, I wanted to share with you, dear readers, some personal insights into our family life when our children were younger. Stephen and I were both physicians, but we struggled, like other families, to do the best we could in raising our children.

As a pediatrician, when our children became sick, my husband would often say I became a "basket case." I was always able to remain calm with my patients, but when it came to my children, I always thought of the worst-case scenario. It was imperative that the children had their pediatrician, Dr. Richard Matsunaga, and he was, indeed, a lifesaver.

As the children got older, accidents were inevitable. Whenever one of our kids or neighbors had minor lacerations that needed stitches, Stephen was ready and prepared to suture anyone in our laundry room. He would lay them on the washer-dryer and always did a magnificent job. Of course, this was a lot easier and quicker than going to the Emergency Room.

Whenever flu season came around, I would take flu shots home to administer to the kids, rather than taking an entire afternoon to take them to their pediatrician. On one of these days, my third son was just not having it, so he escaped and ran outside the house screaming at the top of his lungs, "Why do you want to kill me?" I kept yelling at him to lower his voice, as I thought the neighbors were probably already dialing Child Protective Services. He finally got his Flu shot from Dad when he got home.

As I've mentioned before, parenting is one of the most challenging and underappreciated jobs in the world. When you're raising four "high-spirited" children, challenges would arise daily. I recall a moment when my second son was unhappy about something and yelled, "Why can't we be a normal family?" to which I quickly replied, "One day, you'll realize that we're probably the most normal family on this entire block!"

As our four children grew up, we had our disagreements with them, in addition to the many sibling quarrels they had. Whenever tempers flared, the boys tended to punch holes in the walls or bedroom doors. Whenever this happened, Stephen remained calm and gave them a few hours to figure out a way to fix the holes and later had them write essays on what they learned from the experience. I was always amazed at the ingenious ways Stephen came up with to teach them life lessons. His methods did indeed work.

My husband and I were both physicians, but we never pressured them into being physicians. We always encouraged them to follow their hearts. With two parents as physicians, they saw, daily, the work and dedication it took to be in the medical field. As it turned out, none of them entered the field of medicine, but they have each gone far beyond any expectations I ever dreamed possible.

So, dear parents with children, hang in there and trust God's purpose for them.

"No discipline seems pleasant at the time, but painful. Later, however, it produces a harvest of righteousness and peace for those who have been trained by it. Therefore, strengthen your feeble arms and weak knees."

—HEBREWS 12:11–12 NIV

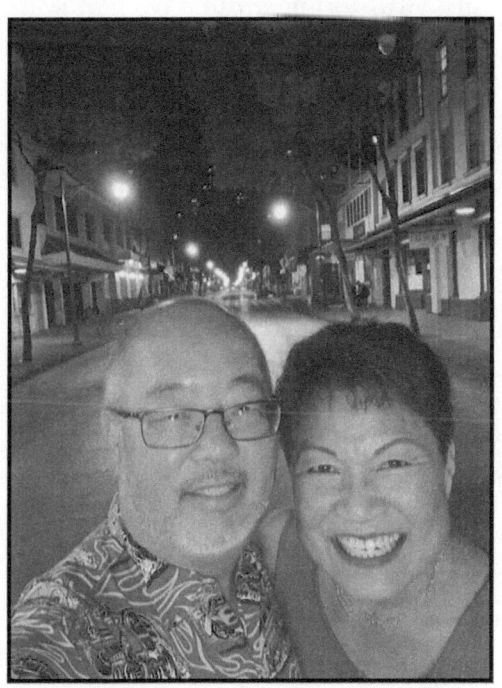

This past weekend, we had street closures in both Chinatown on Saturday evening and Waikiki on Sunday morning, allowing people to gather and support our local businesses. Our Governor is also contemplating a pushback of the opening date of August 1 for Hawaii to reopen to tourists.

If that's not confusing enough, face masks are also advised to be worn outdoors. However, as I drove around this weekend, I saw large crowds playing football or basketball at the park, not wearing face masks. When I go walking, I don't wear a facemask, but I always observe social distancing when I see someone approaching. Sometimes, I wonder if I'll be arrested for not wearing a face mask.

When I tune in to different news channels, I'm fed inconsistent news with a lot of sensationalism and fear woven together in the presentations. Sometimes, it leaves me with more questions than answers and almost paralyzes me in my daily activities.

Yesterday at our church, we discussed the question of "Why is God allowing this deadly virus to linger on?" We had a spirited discussion, and one of the conclusions I walked away with is that this was a battle between "good versus evil" or "God versus no God." I feel the enemy is trying his best to destroy our "hearts, minds, and souls" and create constant doubts, anxieties, and fear in all of us.

But for me, in this time of turmoil, I turn to my God for hope. Just as we all run for shelter when it rains, I will always run to my God as my safe place when things become overwhelming for me. As believers of God, we are all called to trust and serve the Lord. God is involved in every aspect of our lives, and yet we must still do our part to live the best lives possible as believers. God will continue to protect our hearts, minds, and souls, but we are commanded to focus our lives on things that please God. Thus, with a deliberate focus on positive things, we can experience peace through the power of God.

The take-home message during this time of the COVID-19 pandemic, dear readers, is to set aside our worries and anxieties in favor of healthier thoughts. As it is said in Romans 12:22, we are transformed by the renewing of our minds. Let us all replace the negativity that pervades the world's thoughts with the positivity and goodness of Godly thoughts. God wants our minds and calls us to conform our thoughts and actions to His will and His ways.

> *"Finally, brothers and sisters, whatever is true, whatever is noble, whatever is right, whatever is pure, whatever is lovely, whatever is admirable – if anything is excellent or praiseworthy – think about such things. Whatever you have learned or received or heard from me or seen in me – put it into practice. And the God of peace will be with you."*

> —PHILIPPIANS 4 8–9 NIV

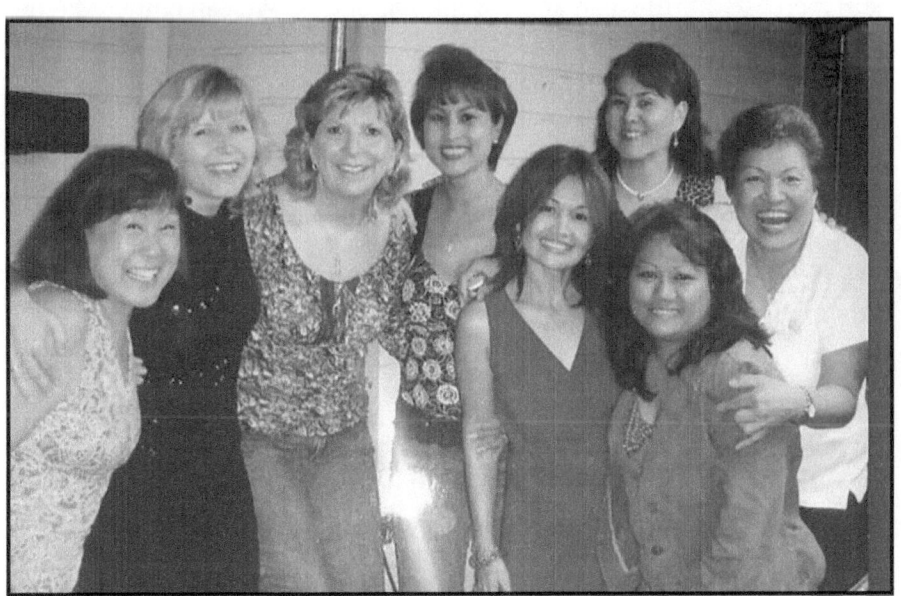

T here have been so many recent studies on the importance of social support and social interactions. There is now evidence that these are two extremely important factors in predicting physical health and wellbeing for people of all ages. Additionally, social support and interactions enhance our immune system, which is now particularly vital during the COVID-19 pandemic. If one lacks social interactions and support, one can succumb to physical illnesses as well.

I recently attended my monthly grief support virtual meeting, and it was wonderful to reconnect with my "grief support family." Even though we can't meet in person, it's refreshing to check in with one another each month. I shared that last month was particularly difficult for me, as it marked the tenth anniversary of my husband Stephen's passing. Throughout the meeting, the recurring word was "family," which perfectly describes how I feel about this group.

Other positive benefits of social interactions are an improved mood and an overall more positive outlook on life, which we all need desperately right now. It can also keep our brains active and sharp, with improved memory. Most importantly, staying socially connected will help increase our lifespan and overall happiness. We can enjoy a higher quality of life with fulfilling social interactions and peers who understand what we are going through.

In 2013, a review of the research showed that "social isolation is on par with high blood pressure, obesity, lack of exercise, or smoking as a risk factor for illness and early death." People who lack social interactions are more likely to experience high levels of stress and inflammation, which in turn can undermine every bodily system.

The bottom line is that for all of us seeking a healthy lifestyle, it is not enough to focus solely on eating our fruit and vegetables or getting regular exercise; we must also remember to stay connected.

So, dear readers, in this COVID-19 pandemic, reach out to someone you know who is isolated, alone, and in need of support. You will both reap the rewards, whether you give or receive the support.

> *"Two are better than one because they have a good return for their work: If one falls, his friend can help him up. But pity the man who falls and has no one to help him up!"*
>
> —ECCLESIASTES 4:9–10 NIV

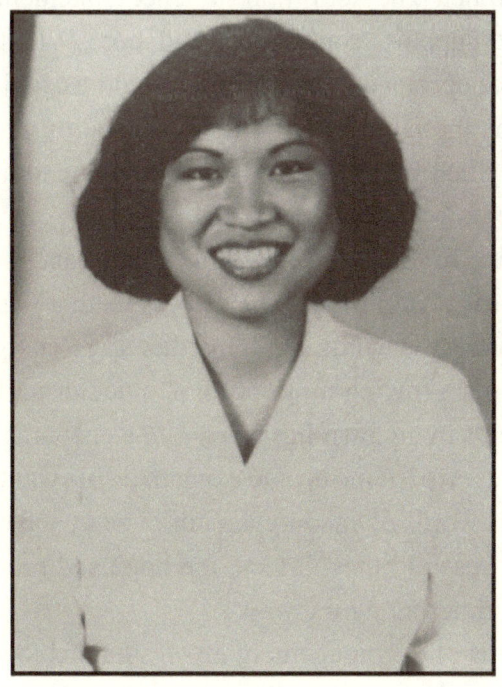

For the past several days, I have found myself doing a lot of "encouraging" to my patients and parents. In part, this seems to be due to the COVID-19 fatigue we've all been experiencing. I just spent an extra thirty minutes giving a pep talk to one of my patients, a high school junior. Her parents both came to Hawaii from China, and ever since she was a little girl, she had always wanted to be a doctor, like me. She now has a 4.2 GPA and has been taking AP classes since her freshman year. Today, she said that the pandemic has given her the time to think about her goal of becoming a doctor. She is now considering a career as a nurse, and perhaps she had dreamed too big.

We had a long conversation, and I encouraged her to continue considering a career as a medical doctor. She has already put in so much effort and grit towards this life goal, and I told her that I genuinely believe in her ability to accomplish it. When she left the office, she felt better and will continue to pursue a career in medicine.

This incident made me pause and think about encouragement and what it meant to her. The definition of "encouragement" is "the act of giving someone support, confidence, and hope." In this COVID-19 world, challenges continue to emerge all around us, and it's easy to feel discouraged. The thought of giving up is constantly present, and there are many times when we think that we have no one to turn to for words of encouragement.

Whenever we're in the middle of a trial and someone comes alongside us to say, "Don't lose hope. I believe that you can do it," it's amazing how those few words can immediately re-energize us.

As a young girl growing up to become a doctor in the sixties, there were key moments in my own life when a few encouraging words from my dad did wonders to lift me up and even made me want to work harder. I always took his words of encouragement to heart and committed them to memory. In stressful times, it gave me hope and prevented me from giving up many times along the way.

For me, words of encouragement always helped to calm me and let me see the bigger picture. I recall getting a C in Honors Calculus my first semester at the UH as a young freshman "pre-med" and going home defeated. I told my dad I quit and don't want to be a doctor anymore. He calmly told me that he knew I would do better next semester and he had complete confidence in me. Well, I did get an A in my second semester of calculus, and I'm glad I stuck it out.

There are many ways to encourage one another. Of course, spoken words can bring healing, but we can also write an encouraging note or a hopeful message on social media. Another way to offer encouragement is to help someone with tasks or be physically present with them. Finally, praying for others can also be a great encouragement to them. New scientific research is emerging on the healing benefits and power of prayer.

So, dear readers, let's all think about encouraging one another. Encouragement gives us confidence, which leads to action, in turn leading to accomplishment, and ultimately to more encouragement.

"You yourselves know that these hands of mine have supplied my own needs and the needs of my companions. In everything I did, I showed you that by this kind of hard work we must help the weak, remembering the words the Lord Jesus Christ himself said: 'It is more blessed to give than to receive.'"

—ACTS 20:34–35 NIV

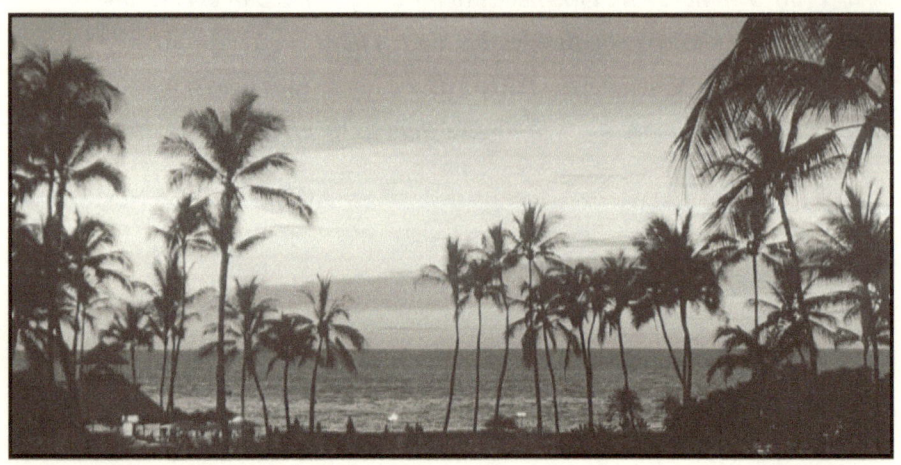

The other day, I got home, and I told my husband, "Let's skip the walk today." Well, he had his shoes on and would have none of that.

When I returned from our walk, I felt rejuvenated and energized, and I thoroughly enjoyed being outdoors after spending the day in the office. The birds were chirping, the sunset was beautiful, the trade winds were blowing, and, of course, I had a great conversation with my husband.

Today, I would like to discuss the numerous proven health benefits of spending time outdoors and in nature. In our beautiful state, we have no excuse, as we have the best weather in the world year-round.

Research indicates that our environment can either increase or decrease our stress, which in turn affects our physical well-being. In other words, what we see, hear, and experience not only affects our mood but also our bodily systems, including our immune system.

We now know that not only being in nature helps us, but also just viewing scenes of nature can help reduce fear, anger, and stress while increasing our pleasant feelings. Exposure to nature makes us not only feel better but also contributes to our physical well-being by reducing blood pressure, heart rate, muscle tension, and the production of stress hormones.

Another interesting study showed that simply having a plant in a room can have a significant positive impact on reducing stress and anxiety. Additionally, nature helps us cope with pain better. There was a classic study done in which people who underwent surgery and recovered in a room with a view of trees did much better in dealing with their pain than the folks who had a room with no windows. (Moral of the story: Whenever possible, get a hospital room with a view.)

When we are outdoors, we start to notice the beauty all around us. Whenever we are with our grandchildren, it seems like we're constantly outdoors. It gives us all a sense of attachment to nature, a calming effect, and allows our brains a break from the everyday grind. In this process, we are refreshing ourselves for new tasks to be tackled later.

When we don't spend time outdoors and spend most of our time in front of our screens, this combination is associated with depression and loneliness.

So, dear readers, especially in this time of COVID-19, let's make a conscious decision to go outdoors daily and enjoy the beauty of our state. It could be as simple as taking a walk, playing a sport, swimming, planting or tending a garden, checking out the flowers blooming, or just sitting on the lanai porch and reading.

> *"Let the heavens rejoice, let the earth be glad, let the sea resound and all that is in it. Let the Felds be jubilant, and everything in them; let all the trees of the forest sing for joy."*
>
> —PSALM 96:11–12 NIV

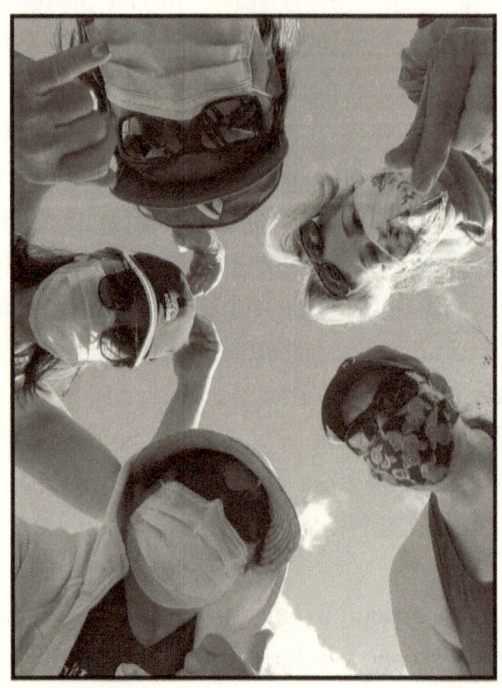

T oday, I would like to discuss the importance of face-to-face contact and its potential contribution to our overall health and well-being, which may lead to longer lives. In this time of COVID-19, everyone wears a mask, and we can only see their eyes. However, even though we can only see people's eyes, scientific studies now show that "in-person" interactions are so much more beneficial than just virtually connecting.

According to psychologist Susan Pinker, when we interact back and forth, we release numerous positive neurotransmitters in our brains, including dopamine. Social interaction enables us to practice problem-solving and engage in person-to-person communication, develop rapport, and connect with another person on a deeper level, fostering a sense of trust. Additionally, she says that humans are a social species and are meant to interact. Studies show that when we are alone and isolated, we die. She named this significant social effect "The Village

Effect," and she has devoted her life's work to demonstrating how face-to-face contact is crucial in making us all healthier, happier, and smarter.

During this time of COVID-19 social distancing, today's topic becomes even more relevant. In 2010, a large-scale study was conducted on over 49,000 people, who were followed for eight years, to determine which lifestyle habits were most predictive of good health and longevity. To their surprise, they found that strong relationships and social support were the two strongest predictors of good health, surpassing factors such as exercise, weight, smoking, and alcohol intake. They also found that not only were close "inner circle" relationships important, but they also noted that the larger your "outer circle" group was, the better off you were. The definition of the outer circle group would be the people you encounter frequently, such as the mailman, the grocery cashier, and fellow employees.

Another study followed over 4,000 women with a diagnosis of breast cancer closely for many years. The findings showed that individuals with larger numbers of personal and social connections were four times more likely to survive breast cancer.

With our current social media, one might conclude that having thousands of virtual friends means you are well-connected and much better off, but the opposite is true. When you are only digitally connected, you're at a greater risk of severe isolation and miss out on the positive benefits of face-to-face interactions. In-person communication is always more beneficial in building social bonds than just connecting digitally. Skype or FaceTime would be a better way of communicating, but they are still not as effective as in-person interaction.

Thus, for inner or outer circle relationships to exist and flourish, we need to tend to them regularly, just as we care for and nurture a plant. If one does not feed it, it will die.

So, dear readers, the take-home lesson today is to maintain eye contact with the people you meet daily and make an extra effort to interact in person. You might just be the one to uplift someone who needs encouragement at that time. Continue to keep increasing your social connections, and everyone will feel better and benefit from it.

"Be wise in the way you act toward outsiders; make the most of every opportunity."

—COLOSSIANS 4:5 NIV

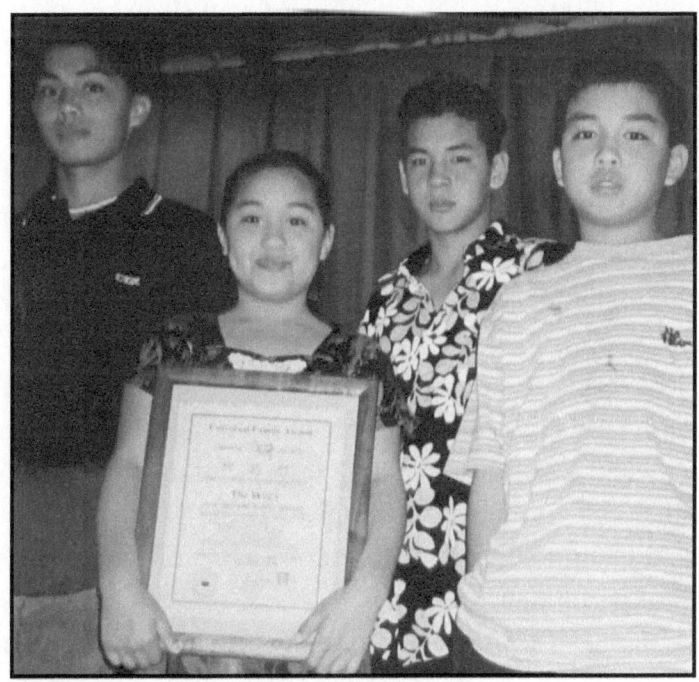

As a pediatrician, I consistently emphasize the importance of exercise and limiting screen time for our children. It is so crucial for parents and grandparents to encourage outdoor play at an early age. Recently, in the office, though, team sports have been cancelled due to the pandemic.

The current recommendation by the American Academy of Pediatrics is to allow young children to try as many different sports or outdoor activities as possible. It could be team sports or individual sports, such as tennis, golf, swimming, hiking, or dancing. By doing this, a child can explore their strengths and weaknesses, and perhaps later, in middle or high school, choose one or two sports to focus on. Another plus to doing it this way is that by cross-training in a variety of activities, the child is exposed to a few sports and subsequently does not overuse or injure certain areas of their body.

When our four children were growing up, Stephen and I always enjoyed doing family activities outdoors. Our weekends were filled with beach outings, picnics, hikes, and many bike rides around the neighborhood. People still remember our family riding around the Gentry Waipio bike paths, all six of us on our bicycles. What a sight that was!

To keep them busy on Saturday mornings, we enrolled them in martial arts classes every Saturday for many years at the "Universal Kempo Karate Schools." They grumbled about going every week and would have preferred staying home to watch cartoons, but we wouldn't have any of that.

As I look back, these weekly martial arts classes were well worth every penny. They might disagree with me, but I felt it made them stronger mentally and physically, instilling respect for their bodies while also teaching them how to defend themselves if the need ever arose. They also entered many tournaments to spar in, which helped them to raise their level of performance.

I think the most valuable part of their classes was at the end when Professor Buell would go over the "word of the week." He would discuss words such as courage, trust, kindness, honesty, loyalty, perseverance, and others. Through their training, classes, and mentoring, I believe they were taught life lessons, even when they appeared disinterested, and these principles have stayed with them.

So, dear parents, consider martial arts, scouting, or other individualized sports, such as tennis, golf, or archery, as a great source of activity for your young child to try, in addition to team sports. Most importantly, allow your young children to have fun while participating in these activities. They will not only cherish these memories for many years to come, but you will also have given them the love of movement and exercise for a lifetime.

"Praise be to the Lord, my Rock, who trains my hands for war, my fingers for battle. He is my loving God and my fortress, my stronghold and my deliverer, my shield, in whom I take refuge, who subdues people under me."

—PSALMS 144:1–2 NIV

ENTRY: 07/20/20

I began writing my daily blogs on March 23, 2020, when Hawaii officially went into lockdown due to the COVID-19 pandemic. I never thought, in my wildest dreams, that I would keep this up. It started as a means of expressing my fears, frustrations, and uncertainties as a business owner, physician, mother, and grandmother. Still, it quickly evolved into a fantastic journey of self-growth and understanding.

To my surprise, these daily blogs have become a very healing experience. It became a means for me to pause and reflect on my day, evaluate it, and seek ways to become a better person.

As I have shared my daily entries with each one of you, my dear readers, I feel that you are now part of my extended family, who have been alongside me on this shared experience. I have genuinely appreciated your honest written and verbal feedback over the past four months. I am always delighted to hear how my blogs have positively impacted so many of you.

I want to encourage you, once again, to give journaling a try. It could become an excellent means to gain insight, healing, and growth. It could also be a way to help solve problems and manage life challenges by simply writing them down by hand and seeing them on paper. In the process of journaling, you force yourself to pause, be in the present moment, and reflect on your life.

For myself, I will be moving on to new projects. Over the next several months, I will conduct additional radio interviews, podcasts, virtual lectures for physicians, and television appearances to discuss my new book further. Even in these unprecedented times of the COVID-19 pandemic, I want my families to know that there is help and hope for them to improve not only physically, but also emotionally and spiritually.

So, dear readers, I will continue to praise God for every day He gives me to do His work. I have been blessed with much and continue to look forward to the new adventures ahead, where I can bless others as much as possible.

"Through Jesus, therefore, let us continually offer to God a sacrifice of praise – the fruit of lips that confess his name. And do not forget to do good and to share with others, for with such sacrifices God is pleased."

—HEBREWS 13:15–16 NIV

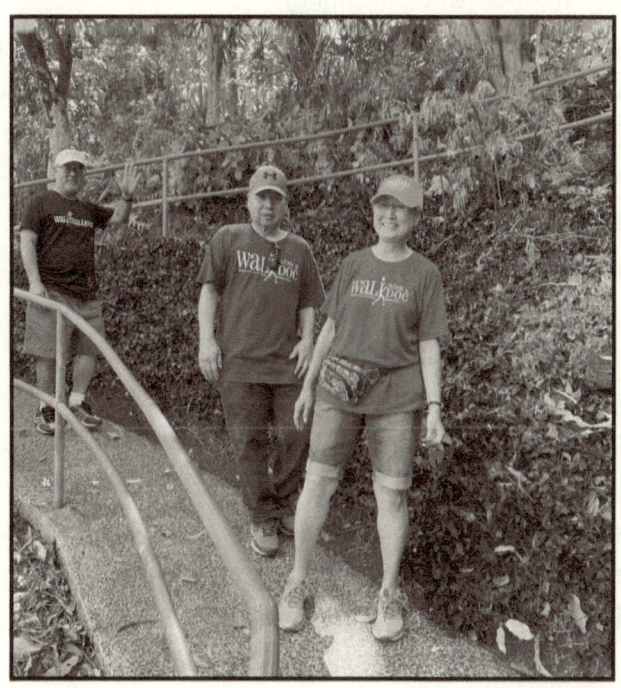

Wow… we dodged the bullet on Hurricane Dougie yesterday! This past weekend was one of hunkering down at home, watching the news on all three local channels 24/7. But then, haven't we all been doing this for the past five months due to COVID-19?

The newscasters kept telling us repeatedly to prepare for the worst and pray for the best. To do this, I tried to pick up a few last-minute items, such as ice, food, and gas for my car, but alas, the lines were too long or the items I wanted were out of stock, so much for my good intentions.

Despite the windy and rainy weather, my husband and I decided to attend church in person. Pastor Jerry's sermon was highly relevant to this challenging time. He told us that every one of us will experience difficult times like these and worse. Since we're human, we'll all have feelings of fear, anger, doubt, and even, at some point, wonder if God is with us or loves us. But he reminded us not to stop there, but instead to go one step further and lay our trust in God, asking Him to draw us even closer to Him in these troubled times.

When we pray for God's protection, He will sometimes shield us from problems. However, there are also times when He allows us to go through tough times, so that we may be strengthened to continue doing the work for which we are destined.

By leaning into God, He promises that we will experience His peace, regardless of our circumstances. As I grow older, I see that it is in the darkest chapters of our lives where He gives us our most significant opportunities for growth and learning. No matter what we are facing, we must lay our faith and trust in God. As the Bible says in Hebrews 11:1, "Now, faith is the substance of things hoped for, the evidence of things not seen."

As we apply faith to our daily lives, we know that any outstanding achievement ever accomplished in this world had to start with someone having faith, even as small as a mustard seed.

My call to action for you, dear readers, is to reflect on the many moments of hardship you have experienced or are currently facing in your life and view them as opportunities to grow, learn, and fulfill the purpose in life that God has destined for you.

Remember, we must all walk by faith in God, not by sight... let us all resolve to be persistent on our path toward our life purpose. Since faith is a gift, it is given to us; all we must do is believe it's ours and walk in it.

> *"In this you greatly rejoice, though now for a little while you may have had to suffer grief in all kinds of trials. These have come so that your faith – of greater worth than gold, which perishes even though refined by fire – may be proved genuine and may result in praise, glory, and honor when Jesus Christ is revealed."*

> —1 PETER 1:6–7 NIV

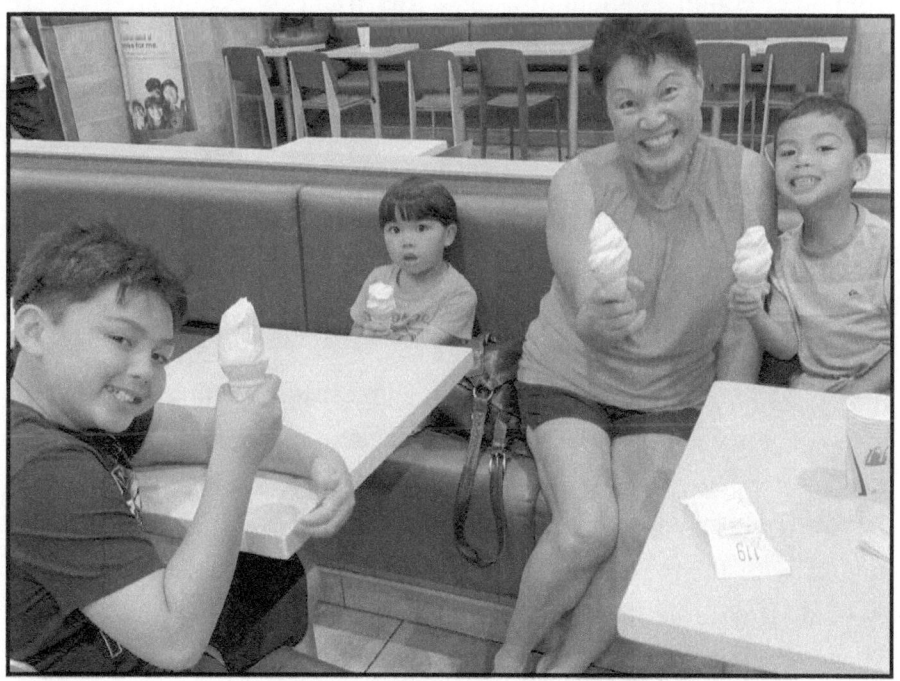

an you believe it's already the end of July? Every day, I await the number of positive COVID-19 tests in our state... it almost feels like my day isn't complete without knowing this number. Alas, the numbers are not looking good and continue to rise.

In my office, parents are expressing their concern and uncertainty about sending their children back to school. More families seem to be opting for virtual school only. I'm constantly getting asked what the right thing to do. The way I answer this is individualized for each family, and the answer depends on the resources available to them, the number of children they have, and other factors.

The current recommendation from the American Academy of Pediatrics is that children are better off in school. They learn best when they are in front of the teacher, but also learn essential social and emotional skills in the classroom. They also benefit from healthy meals, exercise, structured lessons, and mental health support.

Since COVID-19 is a global pandemic, we have learned a great deal from other countries about how this virus affects our children. Here are a few facts:

- Children get infected at a much lower rate than adults.
- Children rarely get severely ill when infected with COVID-19.
- Children don't spread the virus as easily as adults. In households, less than 10 percent of children were the primary spreader.
- The COVID-19 virus spreads more effectively from adult to adult than from child to child.
- So far, there is no evidence to suggest that closing schools will control the transmission of the virus.

So, if you have children or grandchildren, please share this information with them. We can all help prepare them for school opening by being great role models. We can set the example of wearing masks whenever we go out, washing our hands frequently, and always keeping social distancing in mind.

One final note, on this virus and children, is the enormous mental health toll this virus and subsequent restrictions are having on our youth. Suicides in teens are way up, and a rising number of younger children are irritable, acting out, and frustrated.

It is essential to take the time to sit down and truly listen to how they are feeling. Instead of rejecting and ignoring them, be understanding, validate their feelings, and share your views. This is a difficult time, not only for adults, but also for children. Try to remain calm and reassured and let them know that this is not going to last forever. Eventually, things will get back to normal, but for now, we must all do these things to keep everyone safe and healthy.

These are, indeed, sobering and unprecedented times. For me, the only way I get through these days is by laying my trust in God. In desperate times, He wants us to be dependent on him. The Bible tells us again that He truly loves us and promises to help us when we call upon Him. I hope you will trust and call upon Him as well.

> *"My dear brothers and sisters, take note of this: Everyone should be quick to listen, slow to speak and slow to become angry, because human anger does not produce the righteousness that God desires."*
>
> —JAMES 1:19–20 NIV

6

AUGUST

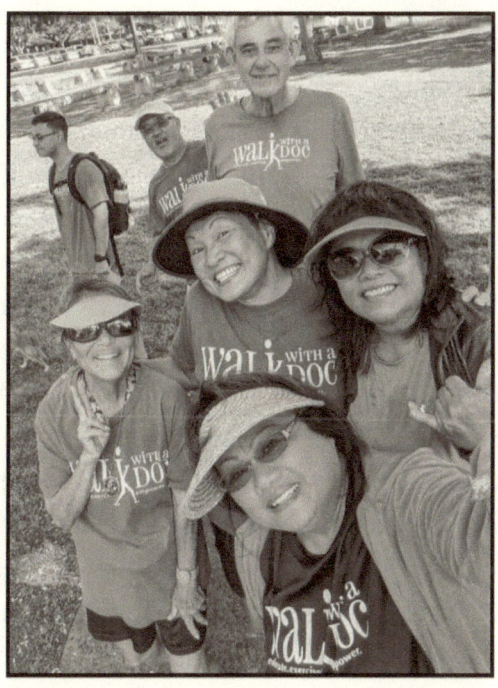

Yesterday, Governor Ige issued a new proclamation, and it was not good news. Due to our recent increase in positive COVID-19 cases, we are reverting to lockdowns.

I don't know about you, but I'm getting extremely frustrated with this back-and-forth process. On the one hand, we seemed to be doing better and slowly opening. I was so happy to announce the return of our weekly Walk with a Doc – Oahu event, and it was great to see everyone once again. However, since city parks are closed once again, we're currently getting the word out on the re-cancellation of our weekly walks.

School is scheduled to start in ten days, and the Department of Education is still grappling with the decision between in-person and virtual teaching. The benefits and risks must be weighed carefully. According to the American Academy of Pediatrics, in a recent statement, children should return to in-school learning for their healthy development and well-being. We now know that some children are suffering without the support of in-person classroom experiences or adequate technology at home.

Currently, children under 18 years make up 22 percent of our population but account for only 2 percent of COVID-19 infections. Worldwide data reveal that children are less susceptible to disease than adults, and they are also less likely to be the primary spreaders in their households. Our experience from other countries has shown that reopening schools has not significantly contributed to community transmission of this virus, provided healthy behaviors are consistently adhered to.

It is important to remember that children rarely get severely ill with this virus and frequently have little to no symptoms. As we age, our susceptibility to this virus increases, making the elderly, who are our most vulnerable population, a priority for protection. However, this virus also throws some curveballs, and sometimes, very healthy young adults can also become very ill. However, as time passes, we learn more about this virus, as well as the most effective treatment methods. We're also getting closer to a vaccine, and if this passes, we will learn more about this virus, as well as the treatment modes, which makes me hopeful.

So, dear readers, I wanted to discuss the *fear* we're all experiencing. The definition of fear, according to the Merriam-Webster Dictionary, is "an unpleasant emotion caused by the belief that someone or something is dangerous, likely to cause pain, or a threat."

We are constantly bombarded with uncertainties from all angles – it's just part of life. Fear can be a powerful emotion that keeps us restricted, paralyzed, and content to remain in our comfort zone. Generally, we're fearful of something that has bombarded us with uncertainties from all angles – the event has not even happened yet, and that makes it impossible to move forward.

In my opinion, the antidote to fear is courage. We need the courage to fight back, stare fear straight in the face, and then push through our fear to move forward. We must refuse to let fear take over and instead remind ourselves that it will all be okay, because it likely will be.

For myself, my courage is my faith. These are very unsettling times for all of us, but I choose to step up and listen to God, my Father. He gives us the gift of love, to support and encourage each other, the gift of prayer to heal our nation, and wisdom from the Holy Spirit to discern the correct actions and feel His peace and calm within us.

> *"All this I have spoken while still with you. But the Advocate, the Holy Spirit, whom the Father will send in my name, will teach you all things and will remind you of everything I have said to you."*
>
> —JOHN 14:25–26 NIV

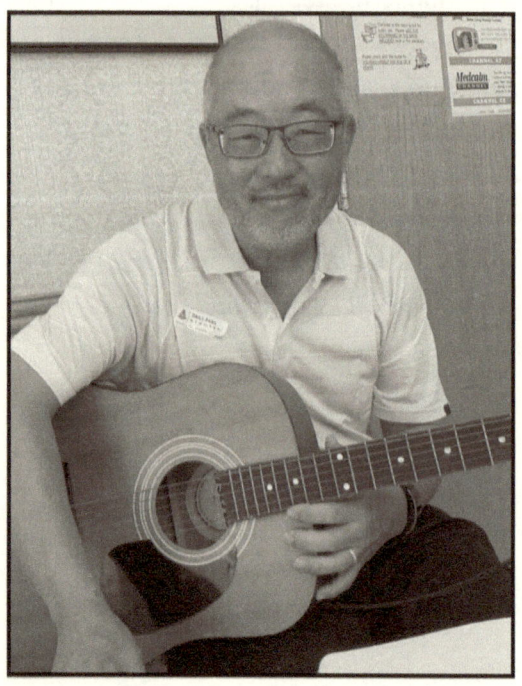

Happy Monday!

When we were driving home from church yesterday, I asked my husband if he was getting bored with the same old routine day after day. Each week, we seem to have the same predictable schedule. There's nothing wrong with this, but our calendars are empty of any celebration or events, date nights out, planned trips for the rest of this year and next year. To my surprise, he told me he is thoroughly enjoying this downtime with me and a season of less busyness.

It made me stop and think that this COVID-19 pandemic shutdown may be a blessing in disguise. For my entire adult life, I've been extremely busy with college, medical school, pediatric residency, marriage, raising four children, and then practicing medicine privately for over thirty-five years. It has been one busy season after another, and I often felt like a robot moving from one activity to the next and never having time for my self-reflection of direction and purpose.

Martin and I will soon be celebrating our eighth wedding anniversary on August 18, and I have learned a great deal from him. One of the main lessons I've learned is to slow down, stop multitasking, and enjoy the moment. I enjoy watching him savor, on our walk, I told him to pick up the pace, but he told me in no uncertain terms that this was not a race and that every morsel of his meals, slowly sipping his ice-cold beer, playing his guitar quietly on the back porch, sitting quietly and watching the sunset, or just reading his Bible regularly. Just the other day, on our walk, I told him to pick up the pace, but he told me in no uncertain terms that this was not a race and that he was enjoying the beautiful sunset. Wow, how do you respond to that?

My first day of medical school is permanently etched in my mind, as Dean Terrence Rogers walked up to the podium and welcomed our new class. He started with something I was not expecting: "Don't forget to smell the flowers along the way." He went on to say that it was vital for each of us to live each day to the fullest. He urged us not to put off important things until later... after residency, after becoming established in practice, or after retirement... because before you know it, your life will be over, and you will regret not having done the important stuff.

So today, I decided to move forward and focus more on the here and now and not get distracted by all the other outside distractions that I have no control over. I am going to use this forced lockdown time to quiet myself each day, reflect on my relationship with God, my life purpose, and the direction I want to take.

So, the take-home lesson, dear readers, is to use this lockdown time for daily self-reflection. Let's all stop being so busy and instead take time to be with our thoughts and thank our Heavenly Father for the many blessings He continues to pour over us.

> *"Search me, God, and know my heart; test me and know my anxious thoughts. See if there is any offensive way in me and lead me in the way everlasting."*

—PSALM 139:23–24 NIV

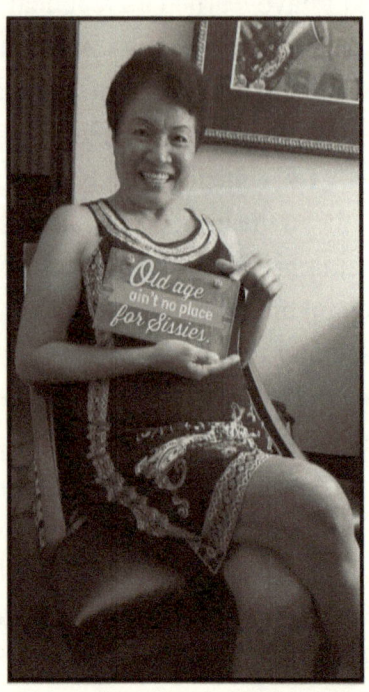

Greetings readers! COVID-19 continues to occupy a great deal of the news time. I even heard suggestions that our Department of Health officials may need to be replaced. I want to remind everyone that this pandemic is uncharted territory. Instead of pointing fingers, we all need to take a deep breath, reassess, and provide the necessary resources so they can do their jobs properly.

Last night, on our sunset stroll, I reflected on my upcoming sixty-sixth birthday and the fact that I'm considered high risk for COVID-19 due to my "advanced" age. Every day at work, I feel blessed to be able to serve our patients, but there is always that little voice saying today is the day you might get this invisible infection. This quiet voice sits in the back of my head, wherever I am.

I recently came across an interesting article that I wanted to share with you. This article comes from England and concludes that people reacted in three distinct ways to the coronavirus:

- The Accepting Group (48 percent): Key characteristics were 87 percent following lockdown rules nearly all the time, only 12 percent reported losing sleep, 8 percent feeling anxious or depressed, felt less likely to lose their job or experience financial difficulties, 73 percent trusted the government's handling of the crisis and only 48 percent checked social media every day – the lowest of the three groups.
- The Suffering Group (44 percent): Key characteristics were 93 percent feeling anxious or depressed since lockdown, 64 percent have slept less or worse than usual, spent much more time thinking of the virus than any of the other groups, 93 percent following lockdown rules nearly all the time (highest of all groups), 70 percent believe that the government acted too slowly, and 64 percent checked social media for updates daily or more frequently. The Resisting Group (9 percent): Only 49 percent say they're complying with lockdown rules, only 55 percent agree that too much fuss is being made of this virus, 41 percent are going against official guidance of meeting with others outside the home, expecting there will be a quick resolution to the viruses and 66 percent check social media daily or more frequently.

Dare I ask, which category do you identify with? I want to think that I'm part of the accepting group. I feel as though I've been in all three categories at one time or another, but after months of this, I've now accepted this and will do what I can to be part of the solution.

I think we can all agree that this current pandemic is confusing, frightening, and unpredictable for all of us. I believe the panic and fear we're experiencing is not from God and keeps pulling us away from Him. Instead, Jesus says many times in the Bible, "Do not be afraid." This is the voice of God that we should listen to and feel the calm and hope that accompany it.

This pandemic appears to be here for a while, so I will continue to take the necessary precautions, help others where I can, and continue to pray daily. I trust that God is always with us and understands our fears and worries. I believe we will move through this together, with God's help. *Chin up, Buttercup!*

> *"Because of the Lord's great love, we are not consumed for his compassions never fail. They are new every morning; great is your faithfulness. I say to myself, 'The Lord is my portion: therefore, I will wait for him.' The Lord is good to those whose hope is in him, to the one who seeks him; it is good to wait quietly for the salvation of the Lord."*
>
> —LAMENTATIONS 3:22–26 NIV

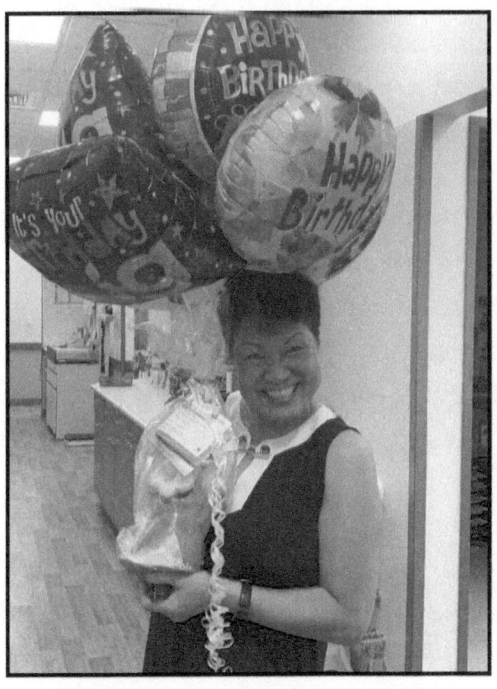

was planning on keeping my birthday low-key today, but it's not turning out that way. First, my husband has been treating me to an entire "birthday week" of surprises! Today, I've had visitors dropping off food and flowers at my office.

I just wanted to thank everyone for all their birthday greetings. I am feeling the love from all of you and know I am a very blessed woman. I thank my heavenly Father for showing me His grace, and I give Him all the glory and praise.

During this COVID-19 pandemic, it is hard to celebrate together, so I have two requests for you to help me celebrate this "momentous" occasion.

I promise, it will only take a few seconds to do, and it will not only reduce your stress, but also support your immune system, improve your mood, and relieve physical tension. Okay, are you ready for it?

The first request is: Make a big smile and laugh!

Yep, that's it, folks. Scientific studies have even proven it to be an effective way to care for both your physical and mental health.

Ready for your next assignment?

Once you've had a good smile and laugh, stand up and do a "happy dance" for me! Yes, just free dance it... nobody is looking at you.

My office staff teases me about this because, for many years, I had a Friday afternoon tradition of doing my "happy dance" once the last patient was seen. It just made me feel good to end my week on this positive note. Try it and you might also like it!

Dear readers, please complete the above assignments and join me in celebrating my birthday party today!

Sending my love and virtual hug to all of you.... Stay safe and healthy.

"Hear, O Lord, and be merciful to me. Lord, be my help.' You have turned my wailing into dancing; you removed my sackcloth and clothed me with joy, so that my heart may sing your praises and not be silent. Lord my God, I will praise you forever."

—PSALM 30:10–12 NIV

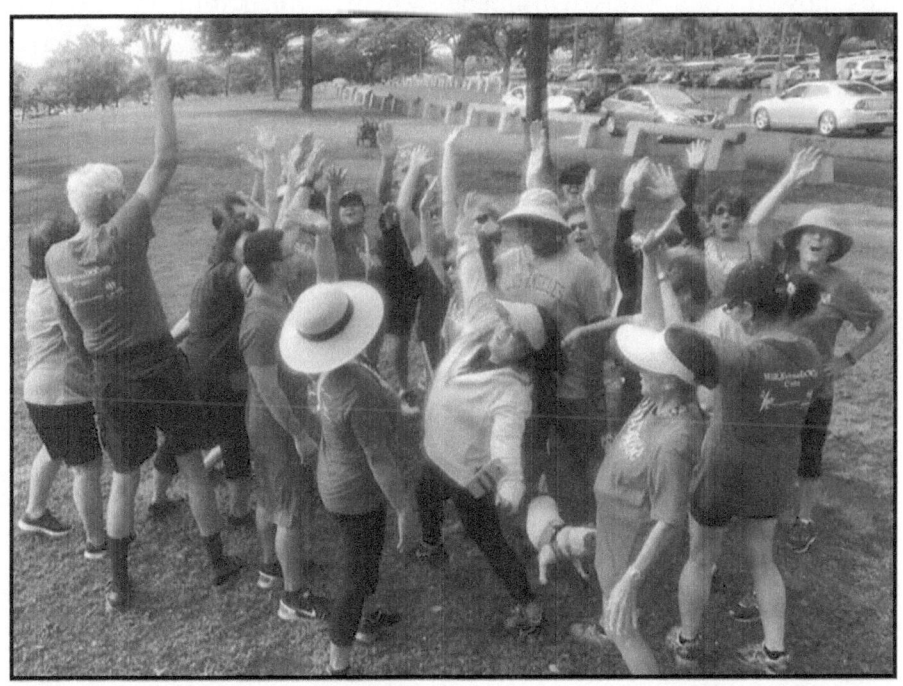

appy Monday, everyone!

Yesterday's front-page headline summarizes how we're all feeling: "Frustration Mounts." This weekend, I read about protests at Honolulu Hale, more small business closures, increased unemployment, extended virtual learning at our schools, as well as a continued fourteen-day quarantine for visitors, among other developments. Times are tough right now. Martin and I even found out the other day that one of our favorite restaurants, Dot's in Wahiawa, had shut down.

For the past six months, we have been repeatedly reminded to wear our face masks, wash our hands, and maintain social distance. With the fun season approaching, these practices have never been more crucial. Depending on whether we heed this advice, we could either see a record drop in fun cases or a never-before-seen dual virus pandemic, with serious consequences. There are already reports that people contract both viruses simultaneously from around the world.

There are still many unknowns about COVID-19, and we're not sure how a compromised immune system from getting the flu will handle a simultaneous COVID-19 infection. Both the flu and COVID-19 are contagious respiratory illnesses caused by two different viruses. Because many of their symptoms are similar, testing is the only accurate way to confirm a diagnosis.

Both the flu and COVID-19 symptoms can vary in severity, ranging from no symptoms to severe ones. Common symptoms of both are fever, cough, difficulty breathing, fatigue, sore throat, runny or stuffy nose, muscle aches, headaches, and vomiting or diarrhea. Differences in presenting symptoms in COVID-19 may include changes in or loss of taste or smell.

Both the flu and COVID-19 are primarily spread through droplets when an infected person, without a mask, sneezes, coughs, or talks in proximity. It is also possible to get either virus by human contact, such as shaking hands or hugging, or by touching surfaces or objects that have the live virus on them. COVID-19 now appears to be more contagious than the flu virus and seems to spread more easily among large gatherings in a short period.

Currently, the most important thing you can do for yourself, and your family is to get the flu vaccine as soon as possible. Medical experts remind us that the flu vaccine is a "dead vaccine," and thus, it is impossible to "catch" the flu from this vaccine. It is very safe and may even save your life.

So, dear readers, we can never be sure what's coming our way in the future; remember that the only thing we have control over is today. Nick Vujcic, who is a well-known speaker born with no arms and legs, is quoted as saying,

> "Take one day at a time. Embrace the positive attitudes, principles, and truths, and you, too, will overcome."

When we get up each morning, it means a new twenty-four hours. Each day means everything's possible again. We live in the moment, die in the moment, and take it all one moment at a time, so pay attention to the present. Smile, breathe, and be grateful for the day… it won't always be this overwhelming.

> *"Never be lacking in zeal, but keep your spiritual fervor, serving the Lord. Be joyful in hope, patient in affection, faithful in prayer. Share with God's people who are in need. Practice hospitality. Bless those who persecute you; bless and do not curse. Rejoice in hope, be patient in tribulation, be constant in prayer."*
>
> —ROMANS 12:11–14 NIV

7

SEPTEMBER

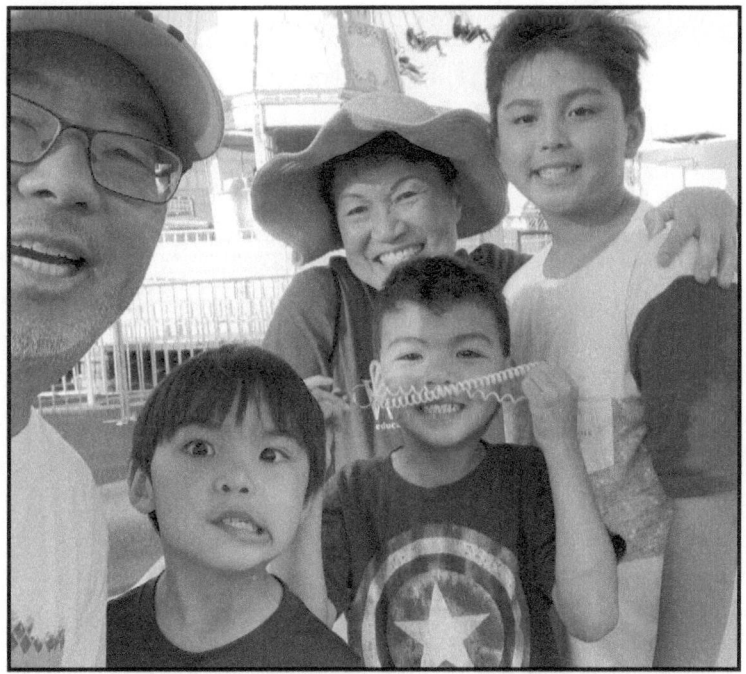

was recently thinking about this pandemic and how it has affected every single person in the world. As a suggestion from my pastor, I recently drew up two columns into "good" and "not-so-good" categories: This is what I came up with:

- I was suddenly forced to social distance, but I'm still alive, not hospitalized, or seriously ill, like so many other seniors.
- I had to reduce my office hours, but I am still employed and able to keep my doors open.
- I miss going out to eat a nice meal, but I'm not starving and have plenty to eat.
- I've had to cancel several trips this year, but this gives me even more to look forward to in the years to come.

What I have concluded from this exercise is that there is always something positive to be thankful for. What about you? Can you not find things in your life right now for which to give thanks and praise to God?

> *"Know that the Lord is God. It is he who made us, and we are his; we are his people, the sheep of his pasture. Enter his gates with thanksgiving and his courts with praise; give thanks to him and praise his name. For the Lord is good and his love endures forever; his faithfulness continues through all generations."*
>
> —PSALM 100:3–5 NIV

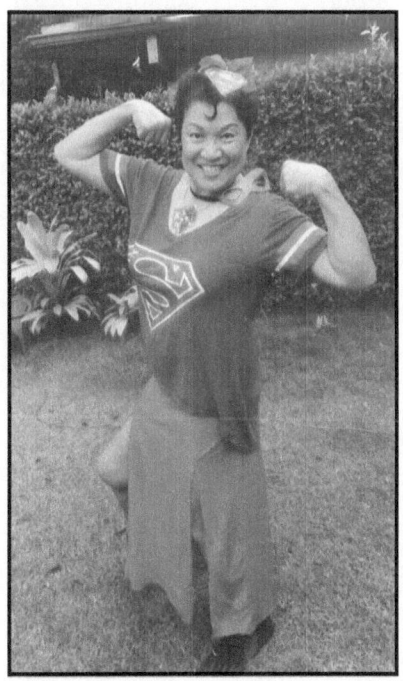

COVID-19 is still with us, and although we're in total lockdown for three more days, the news looked brighter with only 105 new coronavirus cases statewide yesterday. I believe this is the lowest it has been in a while. Today, I want to share with you an inspiring TED Talk by a "Resilience Expert," Dr. Lucy Hone.

You see, not only is she a "resilience expert," but she has used these techniques herself to help her live and grieve, at the same time, when her teenage daughter died tragically in a car accident. In her talk, she shared three practical strategies that I think everyone can use.

In Dr. Hone's words, these strategies allowed her to be an active and resilient participant in navigating through one of the most challenging times in her life. So, dear readers, here are the three strategies to help us deal not only with the coronavirus pandemic, but also with our challenges and tragedies.

Resilient people understand that suffering and tough times are just a part of life. This is a part of every person's human experience. Instead of feeling entitled or immune to the bad things that happen, it's essential to accept that bad things do happen, but also to recognize that we each have a choice to either rise above or sink.

Resilient people choose very carefully where they decide to put their focus. They focus on things that they can change rather than those that they cannot. For those things they cannot change, they leave them alone. You see, our brains are hard-wired to hold onto our negative emotions, like Velcro. However, we must make a conscious effort to recognize the positive feelings that come our way and not let them slip off us, like Teflon. The practical way of doing this is to set aside time every day to think or write down three good things that happened to you. Studies have now shown that regularly practicing this exercise for six months or longer can lead to increased happiness, greater gratitude, and a reduction in depression.

Resilient people ask this crucial question: "Is what I am doing helping or harming me?" Another way of asking the question is, "Is this the best way for me to think or act to get me back on the path to recovery?" When we ask ourselves this question, it immediately puts us back in the driver's seat to make the wisest choices that help us recover, while also being kind to ourselves.

Life isn't always going to be easy, but it shouldn't always be hard. Let's all continue to learn to let go and adapt to change while developing more resilience along the way.

Christ always reminds us that we will face difficult times, but He also assures us that He will always be with us. If He's always with us, then He will help us. Let's all be strong in Him and seek peace by keeping our minds on Him.

"Finally, be strong in the Lord and in his mighty power. Put on
the full armor of God, so that you can take your stand against
the devil's schemes. For our struggle is not against the flesh and

blood, but against the rulers, against the authorities, against the powers of this dark world and against the spiritual forces of evil in the heavenly realms. Therefore, put on the full armor of God so that when the day of evil comes, you may be able to stand your ground, and after you have done everything, to stand."

—EPHESIANS 6:10–13 NIV

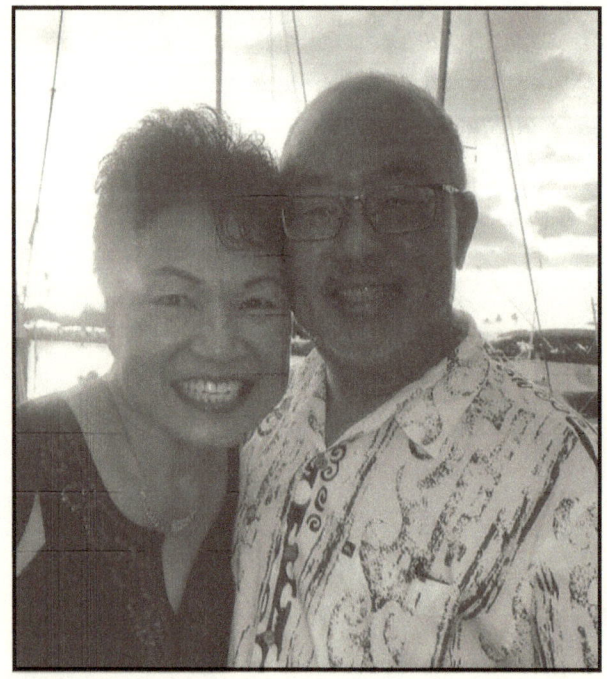

Today we remember 9/11. Where were you nineteen years ago on this fateful day? Today, as an American citizen, I pause to remember the lives of those who died in this tragedy, as well as the heroes who came to help.

For a moment, we all came together as a nation – united, strong, and determined not only to survive, but overcome this evil deed. In the same way, we should remind ourselves during this COVID-19 pandemic that working in harmony makes us all stronger and wiser in overcoming this killer virus.

On September 11, 2001, I think most of us can remember exactly where we were and what we were doing. I remember waking up on that Tuesday morning to prepare breakfast. I turned on the television and to my horror, I saw the live news reports and replays of a plane crashing into Tower One. I couldn't believe my eyes, and soon our entire family gathered to watch the events unfold.

I remember saying a prayer for the people trapped in the towers and what their loved ones must have been feeling. What would I have done in that situation, either as a victim trapped in the tower or a loved one watching this all unfold on live TV? Would I remain on the tower and await help, or would I jump? Would I try to call my loved ones and say goodbye? What would I say in these last moments of my life?

Suddenly, you start to realize what is truly important in your life… and I just hugged my family close that morning. It has been nineteen years now since this national tragedy, but I will never forget that day of September 11, 2001.

I recently visited the 911 Memorials, both in New York City and in Shanksville, Pennsylvania. Each time I think about these visits, I feel sad for the senseless loss of lives, but I also think the courage of the American citizens who did what they could to help one another.

Please do not forget September 11, 2001, and in this time of national turmoil and a deadly pandemic, let us unite as a country and know that *together we can conquer anything.*

God calls his people to live in unity, so it is essential to make every effort to live in harmony, regardless of differences or beliefs. God commands us to do all in love, and it's our responsibility to lead the way, as Christians, toward unity among all nations and people.

My prayer today is "Dear Heavenly Father, I ask that you surround our country with your mighty Hand. Keep us united and help us stand together, living our days with compassion, love, and grace. Amen."

> *"I appeal to you, brothers and sisters, in the name of the Lord Jesus Christ, that all of you agree with one another in what you say and that there be no division among you, but that you be perfectly united in mind and thought."*
>
> —1 CORINTHIANS 1:10 NIV

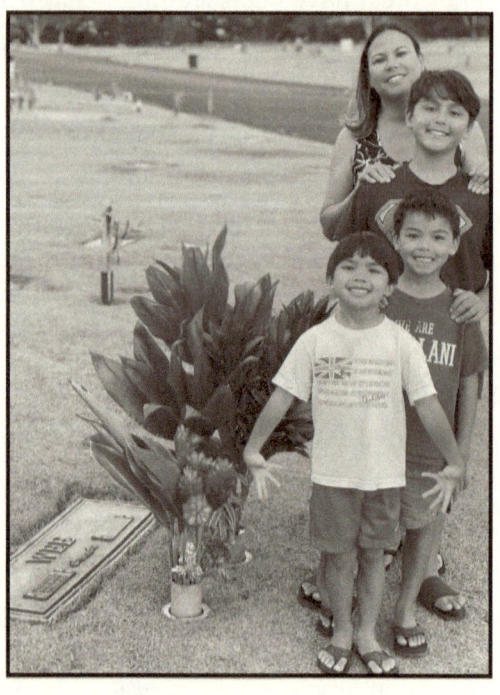

Happy Monday, dear readers!

Today I'm sending thoughts and prayers to a dear friend and fellow physician, Lt. Governor Josh Green, who was recently diagnosed with COVID-19. Please join me and pray for his speedy and complete recovery.

Today, I wanted to share some insights I gained from my virtual monthly grief support group meeting, which was held yesterday. The friends I've made here continue to be a source of comfort and healing, but most of all, comrades who stay by my side as I continue to walk through my grief journey. As always, we shared stories of heartache, strength, recovery, hope, and more. One topic that came up was secondary loss, and I wanted to address this today, as it is relevant not only in the loss of a loved one but also in the context of the COVID-19 pandemic.

Secondary losses are defined as the more minor losses that accompany the death of a loved one or any other traumatic event. These secondary losses represent the cumulative impact of all the unexpected ways we suffer because of this tragedy.

As we all try to proceed toward the "new normal," it is essential to be aware of and learn to anticipate secondary losses… otherwise, they will keep blind siding you repeatedly. Examples of secondary losses can include concrete losses, such as loss of income, home, job, or financial security. However, many other losses are difficult to categorize, such as loss of self-confidence, loss of essential milestones (e.g., funerals, weddings), loss of hope for the future, loss of freedom, and loss of the ability to travel and visit loved ones, among others.

As these secondary losses unfold over time, let us all be prepared to acknowledge these losses and their impact. Only after we identify these losses can we fully mourn, adjust, adapt, and move forward.

Times like these can feel incredibly lonely, even when loved ones are around us. Don't be afraid to reach out for help; this is not a time to retreat and avoid all social contact. If it feels overwhelming, consider reaching out for professional help or consulting with your primary care physician or spiritual leader.

I want to conclude with some sage words from the very popular documentary *March of the Penguins*: "They have wings but cannot fly; they are birds that think they are fish; each year they embark on a nearly impossible journey to find a mate. They walk, but they do not walk alone."

"So do not fear, for I am with you; do not be dismayed, for I am your God. I will strengthen you and help you; I will uphold you with my righteous hand."

—ISIAH 41:10 NIV

I t has been a while since my last blog post, and many things have been happening. Oahu is finally reopening after a two-week "complete shutdown," and our mayor has introduced a new four-tier system.

I believe that advancing this tier system, as laid out, will be very challenging because the number of active COVID-19 cases is expected to continue increasing with more testing and the return of tourists to Hawaii. Another reason we'll likely remain in Tier 1 for a long time is that the relaxation of restrictions will inevitably lead to an increase in infections.

I predict we will be going through a "yoyo" cycle of outbreaks, shutdowns, reopening, outbreaks, shutdowns, and so forth, with no end in sight until a vaccine is developed and implemented next year.

Many lives and small businesses are being ruined daily, with thousands of Hawaii residents struggling to cope. As a small business owner, I understand their plight. The virus is here to stay, and according to Dr. Fauci and other virus experts, they anticipate November and December to have the highest number of positive COVID-19 cases.

I say give the people of Hawaii the freedom to be personally responsible for their safety and the safety of their loved ones. We should not continue to be micromanaged and dictated on how to live every detail of our lives.

Of course, there will always be people who will choose to be uninformed or ignore the mandates and laws, but we have no control over this group. I believe that many people will take responsibility for their actions and comply. So, let's wear face masks, social distance, and remind one another to comply and not let our guard down.

Mayor Caldwell, please open Oahu now before more small businesses shut down for good and our entire economy is ruined.

My prayer today is for God to give our city, state, and national leaders the strength and wisdom to guide their decisions, and may they always prioritize love. During this time of crisis, inspire them and speak to them through the power of the Holy Spirit. In Jesus' name, Amen.

> *"I urge, then, first, that petitions, prayers, intercession, and thanksgiving be made for all people–for kings and all those in authority, that we may live peaceful and quiet lives in all godliness and holiness. This is good and pleases God our Savior."*
>
> —1 TIMOTHY 2:1–3 NIV

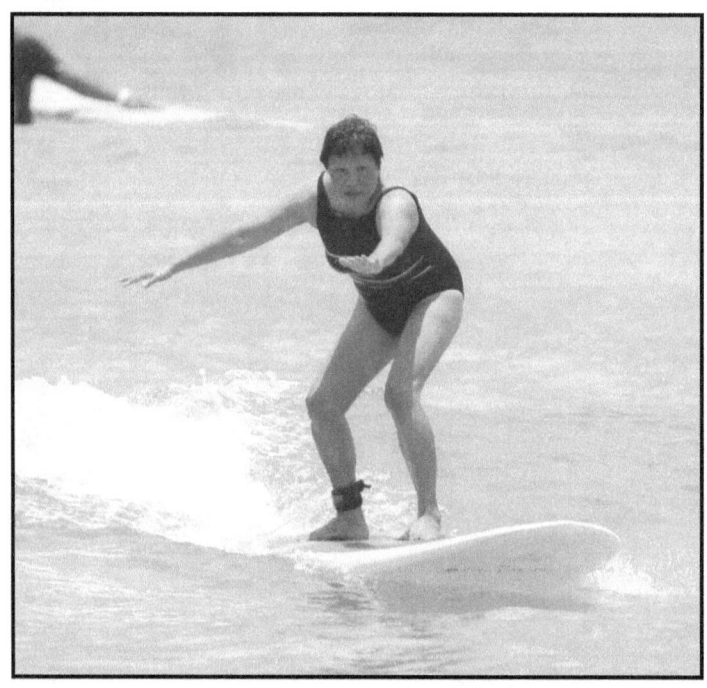

recently listened to an excellent Ted Talk that was highly informative and helpful, and I couldn't wait to share it with you, dear loyal readers.

The talk was given by Dr. Joan Rosenberg, a renowned author and psychologist, who discussed the importance of fully experiencing and mastering our unpleasant emotions. By acquiring knowledge and strategies for handling these challenging emotions, she asserts that we can develop greater emotional strength, confidence, and resilience in all areas of our lives. Developing this skill seems especially important during these turbulent times.

Dr. Rosenberg concludes that what holds most people back in life is not knowing how to deal with these unpleasant feelings. These eight unpleasant feelings she describes are: sadness, shame, helplessness, anger, vulnerability, embarrassment, disappointment, and frustration. When you think about it, no one teaches us how to manage these feelings or handle them, but it's never too late to learn. Once we understand how to move through these unpleasant feelings, we will be able to pursue anything in life.

The formula is simple and can be summed up as follows:

Choice and ninety seconds.

Let's start by looking at the choice. We mistakenly think that our happiness comes from the big decisions in our lives, when in fact it comes from our small, day-to-day moments. Often, when we're experiencing uncomfortable feelings, we automatically run away, hide, deny, shut down, or ignore these feelings. Many of us then turn to food, alcohol, drugs, shopping, social media, or other distractions for comfort.

Scientific studies have shown that once we experience "unpleasant feelings," this immediately triggers our brain to release chemicals that result in physiological sensations lasting for 90 seconds. By learning to "ride the wave" and stay with this unpleasant feeling for 90 seconds physiologically, we will become fully aware of this emotion and gain valuable insight into our feelings. As an analogy, think of the waves coming along the shoreline; sometimes they come calmly, and other times they can be tumultuous. In all cases, they go, linger, and always subside. If we can stay present for 90 seconds, then this emotion will run its course and naturally dissipate.

Pleasant feelings are easy to savor and embrace. However, we must also do the work of learning how to embrace unpleasant feelings in our lives. Life is short, and once empowered, we can set forth courageously to mend relationships, pursue our dreams, and engage in challenging conversations, all because we have learned to "ride the waves of life." Don't be afraid or run away from unpleasant experiences, as this is the key to cultivating confidence and resilience in our lives.

"And pray in the Spirit on all occasions with all kinds of prayers and requests. Be alert and always keep on praying for all the Lord's people."

—EPHESIANS 6:18 NIV

8

OCTOBER

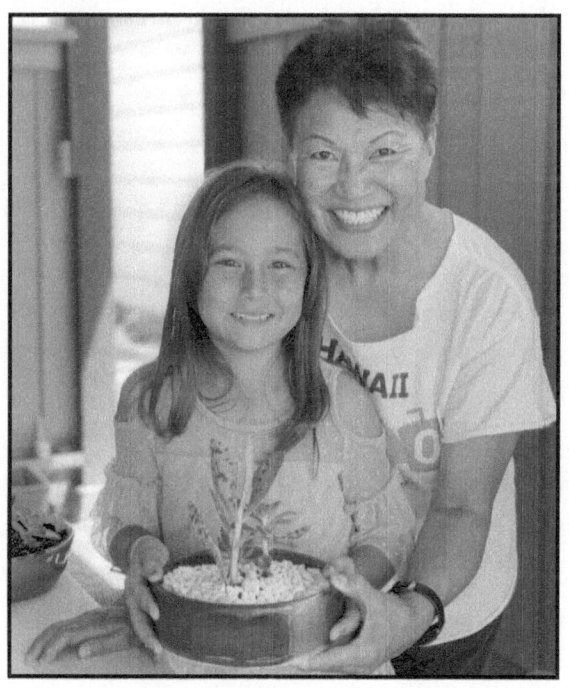

C urrent events continue to make 2020 a year to remember. I'm feeling mentally fatigued, so let's all take a deep breath and pause because tomorrow is not only TGIF but also "World Smile Day."

In 1963, American artist Harvey Ball created the universal yellow "smiley" face emoji. It soon became the worldwide symbol of good cheer and goodwill. In 1999, the first Friday of every October was officially designated World Smile Day to remind us all "to do an act of kindness and help one person smile." In times like these, I wanted to share my thoughts about this with you.

I believe that smiles are buried within each of us, just waiting to emerge, but during these COVID-19 times, we all seem to have forgotten to smile. Smiles are really what we want to see in each other, and they make us all look more appealing and approachable. So even though we're all wearing face masks, we should smile as much as possible because we can still discern smiles through someone's eyes or hear it in their voices.

As I reflect on 2020, the world seems to be filled with numerous complex problems, and there appears to be little reason to smile. Sometimes, it is so overwhelming that I feel too insignificant to make any difference, but I know this is not true. We can each make a positive difference in one another's daily lives. If we send ripples of positivity to one person, they will eventually spread to an even larger group.

Acts of kindness and smiling are highly contagious and will not only uplift everyone around you, but studies now show that they will improve your health and longevity as well. Smiling often boosts your overall mood and lowers your blood pressure. Endorphins, or chemicals responsible for making us happy, are released just by the movement of our facial muscles to create a smile. Faking a smile or laughing works just as well as the real thing because our brain does not distinguish between real and fake emotions. So, smile during those stressful situations, whether you're happy or not, and you'll be able to handle the situation more effectively.

Recent studies also show that smiling and laughing can boost your immune system and increase your lifespan by as much as seven years.

So, spending time with friends and family makes you feel happy. Watching funny shows, making it a habit to smile and laugh regularly, even when you don't feel like it, can also contribute to your happiness. Finally, force yourself to be consciously aware of funny and uplifting things that come your way and be ready to engage in a big smile or belly laugh. Your family and friends will thank you for this, and you will continue to reap the benefits for your body and mind each time.

Remember that our God is faithful, and He will make all things work together for good... so uplift your life by thinking of all the great things He has done for you.

> *"The heart of the righteous weighs its answers, but the mouth of the wicked gushes evil. The Lord is far from the wicked, but he hears the prayer of the righteous. A cheerful look brings joy to the heart, and good news gives health to the bones."*

> —PROVERBS 15:28–30 NIV

ENTRY: 10/02/20

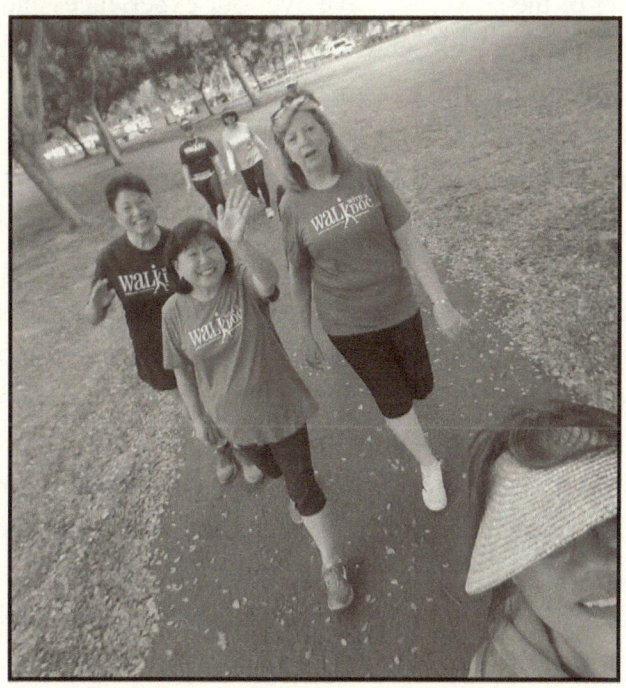

Happy World Smile Day! Today, I am praying for our country's leaders and their staff members for a speedy and uneventful recovery from COVID-19. It doesn't matter which side you are on… let's all come together as a country and wish them well.

2020 has been a year to remember, and we still have three more months to go. When things were improving, we got shut down again. Many lives and livelihoods are being affected; it doesn't matter what age you are. It's easy to feel like a victim amid all this, and as we try to deal with negative thoughts and feelings, we often look outward to place blame on people or events. This pattern is just one way we sometimes use to cope and feel more in control of an uncontrollable situation.

So today, I had to share a beautiful message written by a fantastic friend, Matt De La Cruz. He is the CEO and founder of the Winning Minds Group and is a Certified Speaker, Trainer, and Coach with the John Maxwell Team.

Matt De La Cruz tells a Cherokee tale of two wolves, which serves as a reminder of the power we have over our experiences and emotions. The story is about an old and wise Cherokee teaching his grandson about life. "A terrible fight is going on inside each of us," he said to the boy. "It is a fight between two wolves. One is evil – he is angry, has envy, sorrow, regret, greed, arrogance, self-pity, guilt, resentment, lies, false pride, and superiority." He continued, "The other is good – he is joy, peace, love, hope, serenity, humility, kindness, generosity, truth, compassion, and faith." The grandson thought about it and then asked, "Which wolf will win, Grandfather?" The old Cherokee replied, "The one you feed." (You can follow Matt De La Cruz or get more information about him on: matt@ winningminds.com.)

The lesson from this story is that we each have the freedom to choose which one we want to feed. Do we feed the wolf who is hungry for anger, lies, sorrow, regret, arrogance, self-pity, false pride, superiority, ego, and more? This evil wolf is your inner critic, who tells you that you are a failure, the one who says no one will love you or understand you for who you are. This wolf represents your fears, anxiety, and low self-esteem.

Or will you feed the good wolf? You have the choice to exercise your freedom to nourish joy, peace, love, hope, serenity, humility, kindness, generosity, truth, and happiness. We often look to external objects for our happiness… but happiness is not dependent on these things. Happiness and fulfillment come from our conscious choice to feel this way. So which wolf are you going to choose to feed?

As I reflect on 2020, I'm finally coming to understand that happiness comes from within. I can be happy no matter what my circumstances. It's not the external circumstances that define me, but rather how I react to them that counts. True, authentic happiness is thus my daily choice, one that comes from within.

As Charles Swindoll, a famous pastor and speaker, once said, "Life is 10 percent what happens to you and 90 percent how you respond to it."

"Hear my words, you wise men; listen to me, you men of learning. For the ear tests words as the tongue tests food. Let us discern for ourselves what is right; let us learn together what is good."

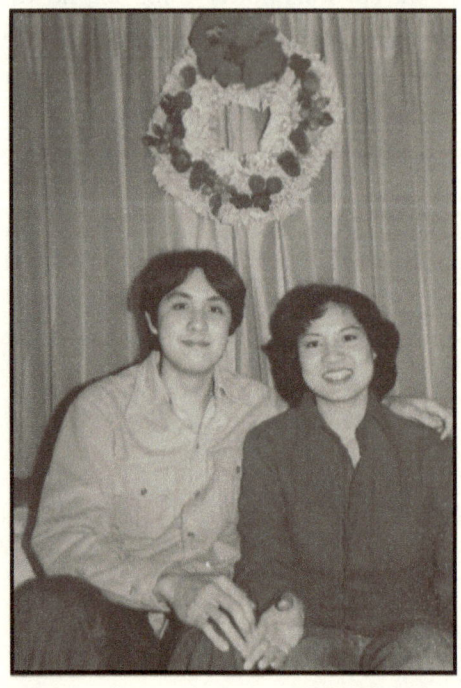

Happy Monday! I recently found myself in a funk... tired of being cooped up, tired of wearing a mask, tired of being careful, and most of all, tired of being told what I can and cannot do. The new term for this is "quarantine fatigue" and our new normal is abnormal. This ongoing, intense stress is wreaking havoc not only on our physical health, but also our mental health.

These current pandemic times have brought back vivid memories of my three years of pediatric residency at Ohio State University's Columbus Children's Hospital. This was probably one of the most challenging periods in my life, and I would like to share with you how I navigated it.

I gained a great deal of knowledge and insight during my first year of residency. On my first night on call, I was on the infectious disease floor, and a nurse came up to ask me what dose of Tylenol to give a patient. I panicked and had to look it up. Within minutes, I was called to help do a spinal tap on a five-year-old boy who died right there on the treatment table with meningococcal meningitis. This is how my first night on call went, and the challenges never ended for the entire three years of training.

The hours were long, and the fatigue was ever-present due to the constant lack of sleep. I worked every Saturday and took night calls on weekends and holidays for three years.

How did I survive these three long years? My husband, Stephen, who was also going through his internal medicine internship at another hospital, was my lifesaver throughout this ordeal. As newlyweds, we rarely saw each other, as our schedules never coincided. However, he would come over to my hospital cafeteria and have dinner with me. One evening, he brought a tablecloth, candles, and a gourmet dinner he prepared for me, and though I was thoroughly embarrassed, I will remember this loving gesture forever.

The other people who got me through this were my fellow interns and residents. We were all in this together, and we rallied together to support one another. We were on the patient floors and on call together, and this was my family away from home. Many of the "attending" were also great. I received encouragement and eventually became dear friends and colleagues. I learned a great deal from these mentors, who continue to be my role models.

The lesson I learned from this experience is that despite the intense and long-term stress, we made it through this tough time by supporting and loving one another. I knew I was not alone, and I cherished every positive gesture and word of encouragement I received during this time.

I know that we will all rise above this COVID-19 pandemic and learn a great deal from it. Things will get better, so let us all hold on to hope and faith in the forefront.

> "Jesus rebuked the demon, and it came out of the boy, and he was healed from that moment. Then the disciples came to Jesus in private and asked, 'Why couldn't we drive it out?' He replied, 'Because you have so little faith. I tell you the truth, if

you have faith as small as a mustard seed, you can say to this mountain, 'Move from here to there' and it will move. Nothing will be impossible for you.'"

—MATTHEW 17:18–20 NIV

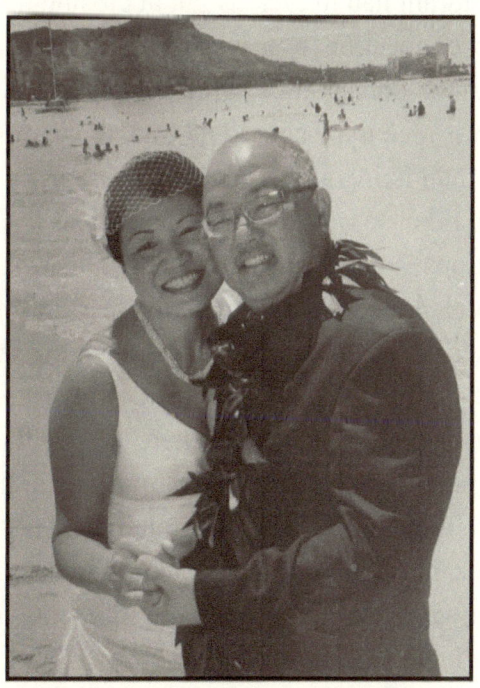

Tomorrow, despite the COVID-19 pandemic, I will be celebrating a special birthday. It will be Martin's sixty-second birthday, and we have a tradition of celebrating our birthdays one or two weeks before the actual day.

When my first husband, Stephen, passed away after thirty years of marriage, I suddenly found myself in the deepest, darkest tunnel of despair that I had ever experienced in my life. It felt like my permanent home, and I was certain there was no way out.

However, Martin slowly changed that. I met Martin on a blind date set up by a mutual church friend. My oldest son told me to stay in public view, and he would be on standby that evening, in case I needed to call him. On this first date, there were no sparks, and I never expected to hear from him again. Our friend, Lori, finally convinced Martin to ask me out for a second date. So, two weeks later, we met, and this time he took out a list of fifteen-plus questions from his pocket. We spent the next several hours answering those questions and getting to know one another. The restaurant had to kick us out at closing that evening.

I believe the connection was instant once we shared our mutual experience of losing our spouses. We began to spend our weekends together, and it was nice to be able to go to a movie or have dinner with someone, rather than being alone. As time passed, we gradually began to introduce each other to our loved ones and dear friends. No one had any major objections, so as they say, the rest is history.

We recently celebrated our eighth anniversary this past August, and this second phase of my life has been just as amazing as the first. Martin has been a great partner to share life with. No matter how crazy my ideas and dreams seem, he is always there to steadfastly support and guide me. He is patient, thoughtful, and committed to the many projects I have assigned to him, and he never complains. I have learned so much from him, but the most important thing he has instilled in me is the importance of slowing down, enjoying the moments, and savoring the precious time we have together.

We don't know how many more years God will give us together, but we're both grateful we somehow met and then took the plunge of marriage for a second time. I have no regrets and wake up each morning feeling so blessed to have this wonderful husband at my side.

So, to my dear husband, thank you for your unwavering love and support. You have been such an encouragement to keep me moving forward in this adventure called life. Happy Birthday, Bud!

> *"And now these three remain: faith, hope, and love. But the greatest of these is love."*
>
> —1 CORINTHIANS 13:13 NIV

Happy Halloween, everyone! Please be safe and enjoy the evening festivities with your family.

Today, I would like to extend a heartfelt thank you to my excellent physicians and office staff at Wee Wellness Center. I have two other physicians working alongside me: Dr. Jordan Arakawa (Pediatrics) and Dr. Lyla Prather (Internal Medicine). Additionally, I have seven other staff members who round out our team. My oldest son, David, is also an active, "behind the scenes" part of the business and has continually supported and guided me throughout these past ten years.

During these unpredictable COVID-19 times, we've all had to learn to be flexible and adapt to changes daily. Despite being a medical facility where one could be exposed to COVID-19 on any given day, my dedicated staff have always shown up to work, ready and willing to give their best in these challenging times.

Everyone now wears a mask all day in the office, despite it feeling extremely suffocating, hot, and uncomfortable. The staff no longer have lunch together in the back room but instead have staggered lunch times and eat at their workspaces. Finally, everyone has been tasked with numerous additional duties, including cleaning and sanitizing the office before and after each patient, to maintain the highest level of cleanliness. Despite these extra duties, I have never heard a single complaint, and they all remain steadfast and consistent with the new protocols.

Finally, due to a decline in families wanting to visit in person, our office hours have had to be adjusted at times. Once again, my staff and physicians have been extremely understanding and accommodating.

I feel incredibly blessed to have this team on board with me and consider them the true heroes who keep the office running smoothly. They work tirelessly, and I'm so grateful to see their loyalty and commitment to my mission of providing first-rate medical care for our community.

So, to my staff, physicians, and my son, David, a great big thank you for all your hard work. Each of you comes with diverse talents and abilities, and I truly appreciate the special gifts that each of you contributes to the practice. This past year will undoubtedly be one to remember, but I'm humbled to be part of a team that has united to accomplish great things.

We still face many challenges ahead in the coming months, but together, with God's blessings, I know we'll not only survive but also thrive.

> *"Above all, love each other deeply, because love covers a multitude of sins. Offer hospitality to one another without grumbling."*

> —1 PETER 4:8–9 NIV

9

NOVEMBER

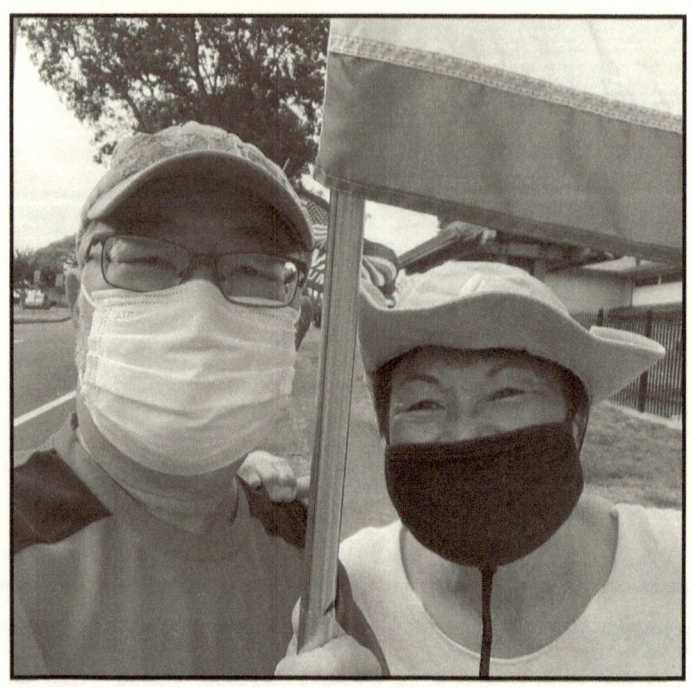

Today is Election Day, and I have no idea what the results of the biggest election of my life will be. Despite the COVID-19 pandemic, the news reports record numbers of voters standing in extremely long lines across our nation.

Here in Hawaii, we were all mailed our ballots, so many of us have already cast our votes and sent them in. However, if you choose to vote in person, you can still do this at selected sites today. The first readout of our Hawaii voting results will come at 7 p.m. tonight. So, hold on folks, we're in for a long night....

No matter which side of the aisle you are on, I think we can all agree that voter fraud cannot and will not be tolerated. I am happy to hear that many key swing states have "poll watchers" from both sides observing the voting process.

Today, I am thinking of our brave founding fathers on this special day. In 1620, a small group of pilgrims landed on this land to establish a new nation founded on the principles of God. They chose freedom, and this is the legacy we must continue to choose for our country.

Ronald Reagan, our fortieth president of the United States, was quoted as saying, "Freedom is never more than one generation away from extinction. We didn't pass it to our children in the bloodstream. It must be fought for, protected, and handed on for them to do the same."

So, as I conclude today's blog, I will leave you with this advice from Rock City Church. Regardless of who wins the presidency for the next four years, let's pray for all our elected leaders, both at the local and national levels. Yes, even if we didn't vote for them and even when they mess up (which they inevitably will). People need to see God's love in what we say and do, so let's keep our identity rooted in Christ and not in a political party.

Go out and exercise your right to vote today.

"Everyone must submit himself to the governing authorities, for there is no authority except that which God has established. The authorities that exist have been established by God."

—ROMANS 13:1 NIV

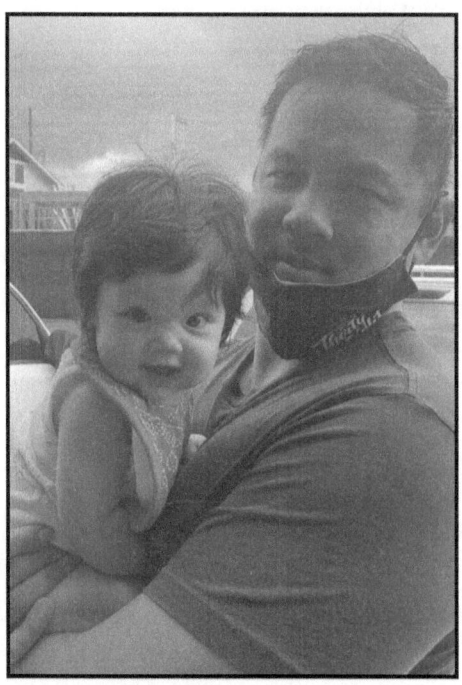

Well, did everyone survive last night? Today is the day after Election Day, 2020, and as the final votes for our presidential race continue to be counted, tensions remain high. America has never been more divided, and I think each side feels so passionately. The great thing is that Hawaii had a record-breaking voter turnout, and this is undoubtedly a step in the right direction. I will accept whatever the result is, provided I feel it was fair and free from voter fraud.

So, dear readers, don't forget to do a little bit of "de-stressing" today. I know I will. Some ideas include taking a short walk outside, taking a few minutes for slow, deep abdominal breaths, drinking water, eating healthy foods, and, of course, getting a good night's sleep tonight. Also, turn off your electronics for a few hours; you don't need to know the five-minute updates of the election.

Last night, my thoughtful husband kept trying to cheer me up. Before we went to sleep, he whispered to me, "No matter what happens, we have each other," and as I pondered this comment, I was able to fall into a deep and restful slumber.

As I look back at 2020, this has been quite a year, and we still have two more months to go! For myself, I turn to my faith and trust in God, asking for His continued blessings on our great nation. As one of my five-year-old patients once told me, when I wasn't having a good day, "It will be okay." I believe that it will, and I will remain hopeful.

On a final note, I want to wish my dearest second son, Christopher Allen Wee, a very happy birthday. You kept our lives exciting and full of adventures. I'm so proud of the loving husband and father that you are, and most of all, the fine young man you have become. I know Dad would have been so proud of you! I am!

> *"Remind the people to be subject to rulers and authorities, to be obedient, to be ready to do whatever is good, to slander no one, to be peaceable and considerate, and to show true humility toward all men."*
>
> —TITUS 3:1–2 NIV

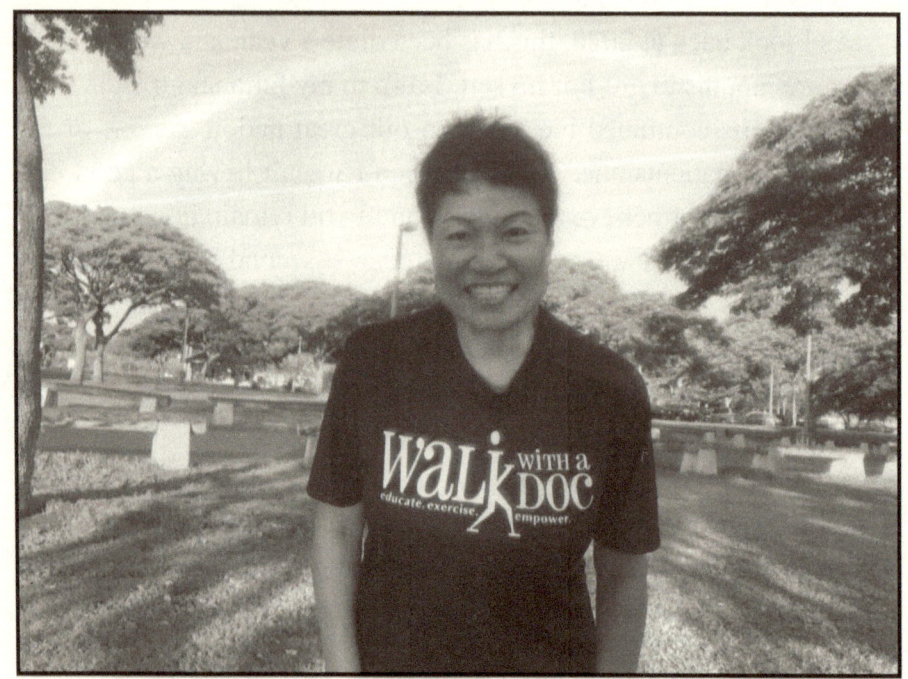

Happy Monday, dear readers! This past week has been very stressful, but life goes on, and I take each day one at a time. An announcement from our mayor recently upset me very much. He declared that Oahu may not advance to Tier 3 in a few weeks, due to our rising number of COVID-19 cases. He even mentioned the possibility of falling back to Tier 1.

My opinion of this lockdown on Oahu is wild. I continue to see the devastating effects of this lockdown on everyone. Not only is it taking a serious economic toll, but a severe mental and physical toll, as well. A recent World Health Organization survey revealed that over 50 percent of Americans are now struggling with significant mental illness, especially anxiety, addiction, and depression. It is now projected that his number will probably continue to rise, even in 2021.

Whenever we are faced with real or perceived threats, we inevitably experience fear, worry, and stress. We also feel anger, but we don't even know who we should be angry at. This feeling of confusion and uncertainty leaves us all feeling powerless.

We have all faced significant changes to our daily schedules and routines. Many parents are facing new realities, such as working from home or losing their jobs, homeschooling their children, or having limited to no contact with loved ones or friends for an extended period. Additionally, physical health problems persist as the pandemic's toll accumulates, and everyone is getting less exercise and sleep.

During this unprecedented time of uncertainty, research is now spotlighting social isolation/ loneliness as one of the significant causes of physical and mental damage to us all. This problem alone is an important public health concern for people of all ages.

So, let's start this new week with some pointers to boost not only our physical health but also our mental health. The following suggestions can help boost your mood and make each day a little more enjoyable.

Make social connections a priority, especially face-to-face: We're social creatures, and we were not made to live in isolation. Seek out the company of others through FaceTime, phone calls, or texting, and see how they're doing.

- Stay active or move more… it's good not only for your body, but also your brain: Any physical activity will improve your memory, lift your mood, and give you better sleep.
- Keep your stress levels in check by scheduling leisure time into your daily schedule and end your day by paying attention to what went well. Every day, take a moment to name two things you are grateful for.
- Practice deep abdominal breathing, yoga, meditation, or journaling to relieve some of your stress.
- Eat a healthy diet: Focus on eating three meals a day, as this will minimize the temptation to snack. Don't forget to stay hydrated with water, especially in Hawaii's humid weather.

- Get enough sleep, as it matters more than you think: Research is now revealing that skipping a few hours here and there can take a significant toll on your mood, energy, and ability to handle stress.
- Find purpose and meaning in your daily life. By making this a daily habit, you will give yourself a reason to get out of bed each morning.
- Finally, seek professional help if you have made consistent efforts and are still not able to function well at home, at work, or in your relationships.

Let me leave you, dear ones, with this Bible verse to encourage you:

"The righteous cry out, and the Lord hears them; he delivers them from all their troubles. The Lord is close to the broken-hearted and saves those who are crushed in spirit. A righteous man may have many troubles, but the Lord delivers them from all."

—PSALM 34:17–19 NIV

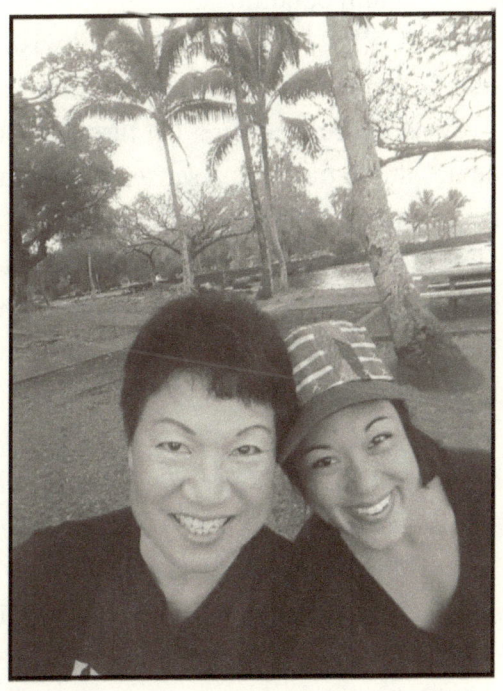

Happy Thursday, my dear blog readers….

This morning, I listened to one of my favorite medical doctors on YouTube, "Z-Dog," discussing the new COVID-19 vaccine being released by Pfizer. He mentioned that preliminary results show an excellent 90 percent efficacy rate. In comparison, the flu vaccine has only a 40–60 percent efficacy rate. However, there are so many more things to consider before getting it. For example: How long will the immunity last? What are the long-term side effects? Will a booster be needed? What about our children, as trials have only been extended to age sixteen?

Then, there is the practicality of distributing this vaccine worldwide. It must be stored at a very low temperature to remain effective, and only a specialized vaccine freezer can maintain this temperature. We must also consider the priority of who gets the vaccine first: possibly healthcare workers, teachers, the elderly, vulnerable minority populations, and those with underlying health conditions.

We're all tired of COVID-19, and I feel you! I wish I could make it go away with a snap of a finger and have life return to "normal," but it's not looking that way soon. Let's all first get through Thanksgiving and Christmas, maybe not in the traditional sense, but we can still celebrate and be grateful for the many blessings we do have.

Due to COVID-19, my daughter, Malia, who lives in New York City, will not be coming home for the holiday season, as she usually does. I'm a little bummed about this, but we've been FaceTiming frequently. Thank goodness for this technology!

> *"Praise be to the God and Father of our Lord Jesus Christ, the Father of compassion and the God of all comfort, who comforts us in all our troubles, so that we can comfort those in any trouble with the comfort we ourselves receive from God. For just as the sufferings of Christ flow over into our lives, so also through Christ our comfort overflows."*

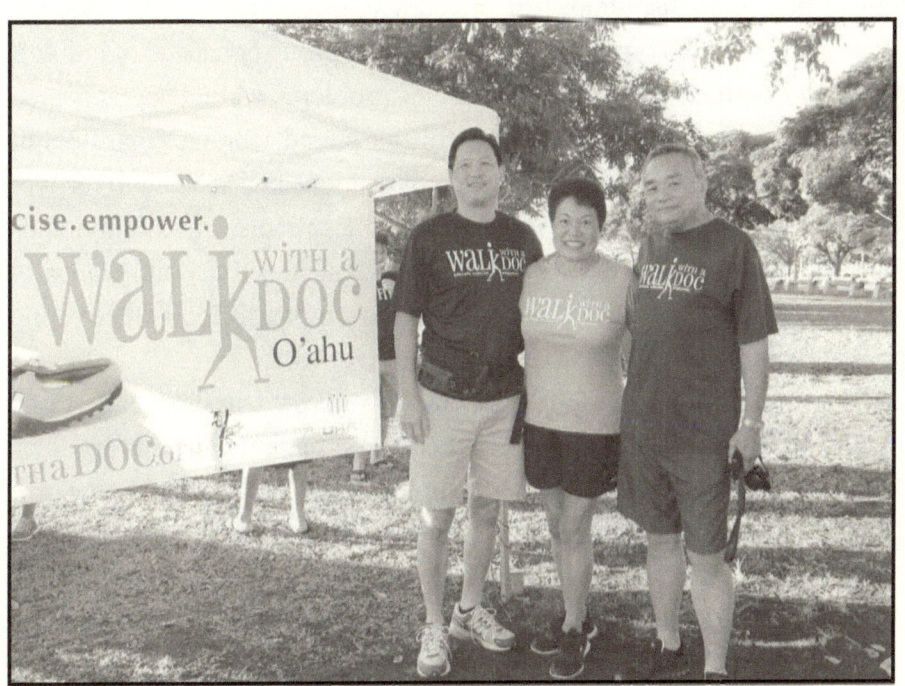

Happy Sunday everyone! Today, I wanted to share with you an exciting virtual adventure I began yesterday through Walk with a Doc. It is the Mount Kilimanjaro virtual 44-mile climb from November 14–28, 2020. I'm taking this challenge very seriously, and yesterday I walked ten miles! I was extremely sore, but I felt a lot better today and logged five miles. The work week will begin tomorrow, so I may not be able to log as many miles, but I will complete the forty-four miles in these fourteen days.

I decided to take on this challenge to motivate myself to incorporate more exercise into my daily routine. This COVID-19 pandemic has kept me somewhat isolated, and at times, I feel sluggish. There are nearly 500 other walkers around the world who have taken up this Mount Kilimanjaro challenge, and we will be connecting through Facebook. It is still not too late to join me or even donate to a good cause. Check it out on my Facebook page.

The founder of Walk with a Doc is Dr. David Sabgir. This movement began in Columbus, Ohio, fifteen years ago. As a cardiology resident, Dr. Sabgir saw two types of patients: the first group consisted of individuals who seemed to manage their heart problems well. They appeared to be very physically active, mentally sharp, and vibrant, regardless of their age. They also had many social connections and seemed to recover much more quickly. In the second group of patients, these individuals appeared to have stopped or slowed their physical activity and gradually lost social connections. They seemed to have more difficulty recovering or improving their health status.

Dr. Sabgir kept telling his patients to walk or exercise, but no one listened. However, one day, he invited some patients to join him for a walk at a nearby park, and lo and behold, "Walk with a Doc" was born! Walk with a Doc's mission is not only to help empower people of all ages to exercise but also to give them the social connections that are so vital for optimal health. Additionally, at each Walk with a Doc session, a doctor provides a short health tip to educate participants as well.

After participating in Walk with a Doc – Oahu since 2016, at Patsy T. Mink Central Oahu Regional Park every Saturday from 8:00 AM to 9:00 AM, I have personally witnessed the amazing transformation that just a little encouragement and regular walking have made for many of my walkers. Although I had to pause our Saturday walks for most of 2020 due to the COVID-19 pandemic, I've every intention of restarting them in 2021 when we get the green light to do so.

During the COVID-19 pandemic, dear readers, take care of your health. I urge each of you to make even a small effort to move a little more throughout the day. It could be as simple as walking the dog, doing chores, or taking a walk with your children or spouse to catch up on things, or something fun like dancing, biking, or swimming. Any movement counts, and I guarantee you'll feel a whole lot better.

Okay, wish me luck as I embark on my virtual climb up Mount Kilimanjaro, and I will keep you updated on my progress.

"For God, who said, 'Let light shine out of darkness,' made his light shine in our hearts to give us the light of the knowledge of the glory of God in the face of Christ. But we have this treasure in jars of clay to show that this all-surpassing power is from God and not from us. We are hard pressed on every side but not crushed; perplexed, but not in despair; persecuted but not abandoned; struck down but not destroyed. We always carry around in our body the death of Jesus, so that the life of Jesus may also be revealed in our body."

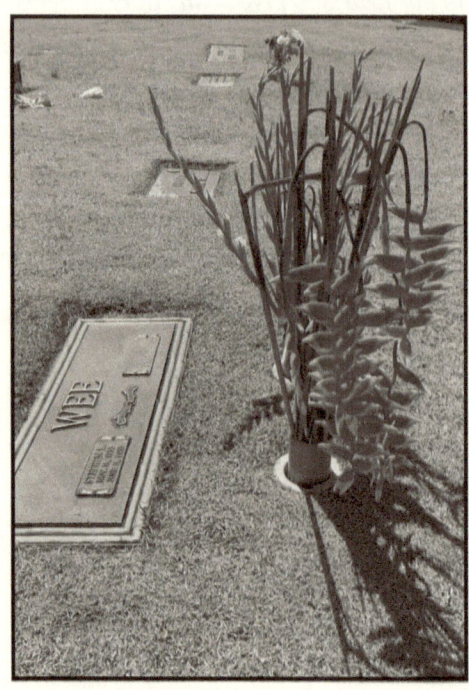

Today is Monday, November 16, 2020, and it would have been my first husband's sixty-seventh birthday. It has been ten years since his sudden and unexpected death, which left us all in shock.

It is so difficult to put into words the deep sense of loss I felt after thirty years of marriage, raising four children, and being together in our medical practices. My world crumbled right in front of me that fateful day, and my life would never be the same again.

How do I move forward without my husband? Am I the only one to feel so lost and devastated? Why does the rest of the world keep going on when my world just got smashed to bits? How did other wives or husbands move on? No one wants to discuss it with me. So many questions and so few answers!

I remember a quote I read early in my grief journey: "Every challenge you encounter in life is a fork in the road. You have the choice to choose which way to go – backward, forward, breakdown, or breakthrough." It would have been easier to fade into the sunset, but it was only through the grace of God, loved ones, and dear friends that I was able to push forward, one day at a time. My grief journey continues, and I now realize it will never end.

There is a short essay entitled *"Love Remembers" by Henri Nouwen, which was recently sent to me* by my grief support facilitator, Pastor J.P. Sabbith. It helped me understand that although Stephen is not physically here, he continues to be significant in my heart and memories. He left a legacy of love, and I hope to continue my life in the same way – to grow in love, receive love, and give love. Mr. Nouwen goes on to say, "When I die, love continues to be active, and from full communion with God, I am present by love to those I leave behind."

Thank you, Stephen, for thirty wonderful years as your wife. As I look back, marrying you was the best decision I ever made in my life! Happy sixty-seventh Heavenly Birthday! I love you and you will always be in my heart.

> *"I tell you the truth, you will weep and mourn while the world rejoices. You will grieve, but your grief will turn to joy. A woman giving birth to a child has pain because her time has come; but when her baby is born, she forgets the anguish because of her joy that a child is born into the world. So, with you: Now is your time of grief, but I will see you again and you will rejoice, and no one will take away your joy."*
>
> —JOHN 16:20–22 NIV

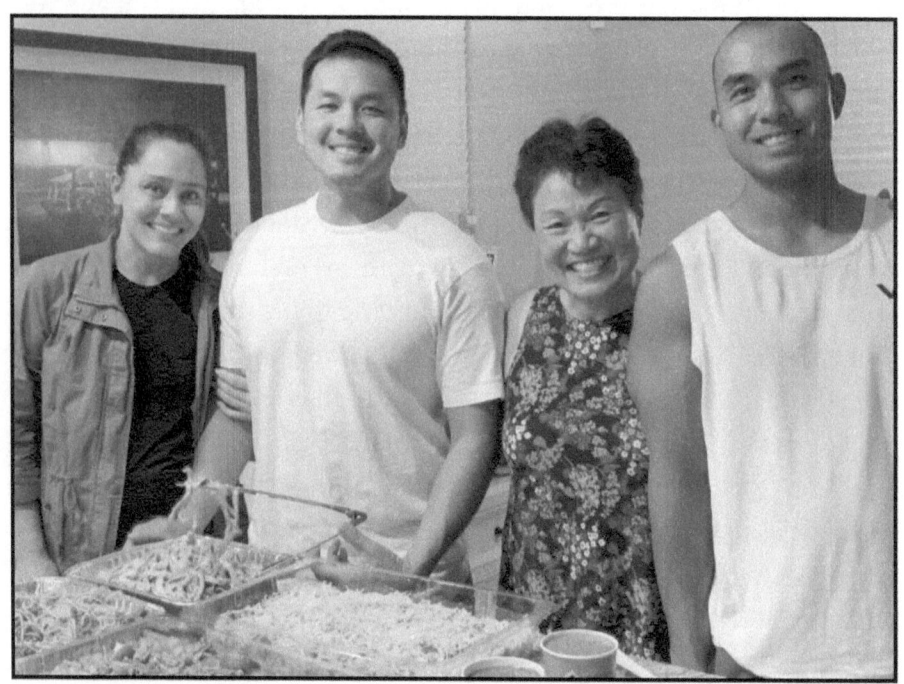

H appy Tuesday! Can you believe Thanksgiving is just two days away? Our local leaders are all urging us to use "vigilance" as the Holiday Season approaches. Hawaii health officials are discouraging multiple households from gathering as they believe this will result in the highest risk scenarios for transmitting COVID-19.

I recently read an article by the head of our Centers for Disease Control, Robert Redfield, who admitted that the forced lockdown is now killing way more Americans than COVID-19. Sadly, we're now seeing far greater suicide rates than deaths from COVID-19. Additionally, there are more deaths from drug overdose than in pre-COVID-19 times. He concludes that pandemic lockdowns are now killing at least twice the number of Americans as COVID-19. The Hippocratic Oath, which all physicians take, has a central theme of "First do no harm." The takeaway point of this is that, in some instances, it may be better to do nothing rather than intervene and potentially cause more harm than good. Perhaps, in this pandemic, it now appears that loosening lockdowns and returning to normal may be the wiser path to follow.

The mental stress and anxiety caused by this virus will undoubtedly end up causing more problems than the lockdown itself. We all know that isolation, stress, and anxiety will exacerbate a host of medical issues, including high blood pressure, heart failure, infectious diseases, and cancer. It seems ridiculous to now see that the cure is twice as fatal as the disease.

On another lighter note, let me shift gears and share a health tip that may come in handy, especially when we approach the holiday feast. According to several scientific studies, it is now proven that people who eat quickly are at a far higher risk of becoming obese and have a propensity to type 2 diabetes and cardiovascular disease.

Japanese researchers studied more than 1,000 men and women (with an average age of fifty-one years) and followed this group for five years. They concluded that 12 percent of fast eaters developed pre-diabetes or metabolic syndrome. In contrast, only 2.3 percent of slow eaters did.

In another study, fast eaters gained twice as much weight over eight years as average or slow eaters did.

Finally, a third study, published in the Journal of the Academy of Nutrition and Dietetics, demonstrated that normal-weight slow eaters consumed significantly fewer calories while feeling more satisfied than fast eaters.

The take-home lesson is to be mindful of how quickly you are eating your meal; in the long run, it could help you keep those pounds off. Here are some practical tips to slow you down, so that your "I'm full" hormone, leptin, has time to signal you to stop eating:

- Chew each bite fifteen to twenty times.
- Put your utensils down between bites.
- Engage in conversation with others during your meal.
- Drink sips of water between bites.
- Savor each bite by noticing the colors on your plate, appreciating the aromas, and feeling the texture of each bite in your mouth.

Go ahead and give this a try, you have nothing to lose… except pounds.

"Taste and see that the Lord is good; blessed is the one who takes refuge in Him. Fear the Lord, you his saints, for those who fear him lack nothing."

—PSALM 34:8–9 NIV

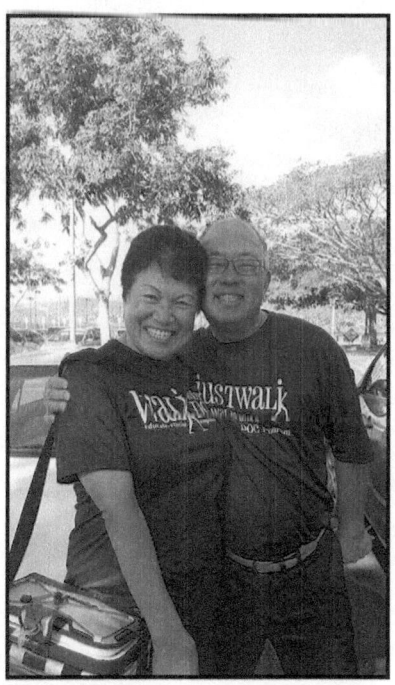

Greetings on this Thanksgiving Eve. I just finished seeing my patients in the office this morning and wanted to write a blog before the *big* holiday. As you are all aware, multiple family gatherings tomorrow have been likened to adding gasoline to the fire, potentially causing our COVID-19 case numbers to rise even more quickly. So, dear readers, please use common sense when making your decision on what to do tomorrow.

Today, I wanted to share an incredible story that our pastor, Pastor Jerry Higashi, shared with us during his message at our Momilani Christian Church congregation this past Sunday.

It is the story of the "black dot on a white paper," and it goes like this:

> A professor surprised his students with a quiz one day. To their surprise, it was simply plain white paper with a black dot staring at them. The instructions were simple: "Write an essay

on what you see before you." They went to work, but this was not an easy task…. They tried to describe the location of the black dot, the size, and its color. After all, what else can you say about this? He collected all the papers, read them, and then stood up to address them.

The professor went on to say, "Did you notice that each of you focused on the black dot? None of you wrote about the vast amount of white paper surrounding it. The same applies to life…. Life is like a large piece of white paper. God has given all of us this life to enjoy, yet we insist on focusing on life's limitations and imperfections, which is the black dot on the paper. Instead of enjoying the good things all around us, like family, friends, nature, etc., we quickly zoom in on the black dots which are issues concerning our relationship, work, finances, etc."

Although the black dot is tiny in comparison to the white sheet, it remains the focal point of our thoughts throughout the day. As we approach Thanksgiving tomorrow, let us reflect on our blessings, the good things and memorable moments of our lives. Always remember to keep that tiny black spot in perspective and instead focus on the white paper.

Martin and I wish you all a wonderful and safe Thanksgiving!

"Give thanks to the Lord, for he is good; his love endures forever."

—1 CHRONICLES 16:34 NIV

ENTRY: 11/30/20

December is around the corner, and it's hard to believe the year will soon be coming to an end. I had a quiet Thanksgiving with my husband, and we thoroughly enjoyed our time together. I missed our traditional large get-together with the entire family, but there will always be next year. I know things will improve, and we must all stay optimistic.

As Christmas break approaches soon, and with the ongoing pandemic, I wanted to share some thoughts once again on the incredible importance of having regular family meals together. Everyone will be at home for Christmas break, so you can give it a try. You'll be surprised at the results of simply sharing meals as a family. As an everyday ritual, the family meal is a symbol of shared family life. It organizes our lives, brings us together, and contributes to our physical, mental, and social well-being. Sharing family meals regularly, whether it's breakfast, lunch, or dinner, has been repeatedly shown to reap numerous benefits. They include improved family relationships, healthier lifestyle choices, obesity prevention, reduced risk of children engaging in high-risk behaviors, stress relief, and cost-effectiveness.

Now that you know the enormous benefits of family meals, make it a top priority. Take baby steps toward this goal by incorporating it gradually into your busy schedules. For example, if you've never had family meals together, start by having one once a week. Remember: the slower any change is made, the more permanent it will become in your routine. Get the entire household involved in planning, grocery shopping, food preparation, and cleanup.

Don't forget to turn off all electronics during family meals and be mindful of the moment without any interruptions.

So, let these small moments at the table create stronger connections away from the table. *Bon appetite!*

"For God did not appoint us to suffer wrath but to receive salvation through our Lord Jesus Christ. He died for us so that, whether we are awake or asleep, we may live together with him. Therefore, encourage one another and build each other up, just as in fact you are doing."

—1 THESSOLONIANS 5:9–11 NIV

10

DECEMBER

Today is December 7, and seventy-nine years ago, President Roosevelt called this day "a date which will live in infamy." We remember, with deep gratitude, the thousands of Americans who defended our country that day. On December 7, 1941, the surprise attack on Pearl Harbor ultimately thrust our nation into World War II.

Since COVID-19 has cancelled our traditional celebrations to honor the great heroes who fought for our country, I wanted to take this time to remind everyone about this important date.

I vividly recall the stories my parents and grandparents told us about their experiences and feelings on that fateful day in Hawaii. It was a beautiful, typical Sunday morning, and the attack by the Japanese was unexpected. Soon after the bombings on Pearl Harbor and other parts of Oahu, pandemonium, chaos, and fear ensued. My mom told me how she and her siblings all ran for cover in their bathtub. My grandparents placed pillows over them in case debris fell on them. Soon, martial law was declared, and all lights had to be turned off after dusk, for fear of another surprise attack. My parents were in high school then, and soon after the Pearl Harbor bombings, school was closed. When school resumed, each student was issued a gas mask to wear whenever they were outdoors.

During the COVID-19 pandemic, I am even more grateful for those who have served and continue to serve in our military. Many gave the ultimate sacrifice and died in the line of duty. I want to do my best as an American citizen to uphold the Godly truths in America's three founding documents, collectively known as the Charters of Freedom, which are the Declaration of Independence, the Constitution, and the Bill of Rights. Together, these documents have secured the rights of the American people for more than two and a quarter century.

Thank you to all military personnel, past, present, and future, as well as their families, for all their sacrifices to keep us safe and free from tyranny. This is the reason why we should all continue to salute the flag, put our hands over our hearts, and stand for the national anthem. What makes America great today is that we will never forget the sacrifices previous generations made to keep our country free.

We are so blessed to live in America. We are not a perfect nation, but we are still the best in the world. We should never forget the sacrifices made by so many and never let our guard down, as there are truly evil forces out there who want to see us destroyed. Today, I pray for God's continued blessings over our nation and vow never to forget December 07, 1941.

> *"As the Father has loved me, so I have loved you. Now remain in my love. If you obey my commands, you will remain in my love, just as I have obeyed my Father's commands and remain in his love. I have told you this so that my joy may be in you and that your joy may be complete. My command is this: Love each other as I have loved you."*
>
> —JOHN 15:9–12 NIV

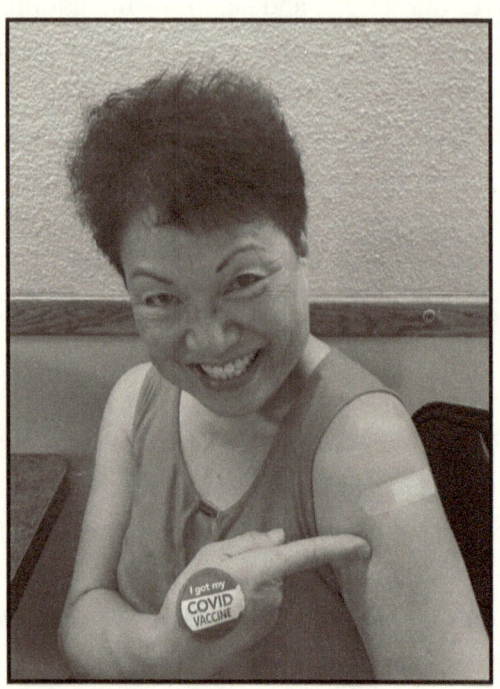

The COVID-19 vaccine has arrived in Hawaii, and I hope it will begin to have a positive impact on the COVID-19 pandemic. As time goes on, we're now seeing that this virus causes some severe problems, which include not only severe chronic lung damage but also thickening of the blood, which results in clots in various parts of the body. Sometimes, this can result in loss of limbs, strokes, heart attacks, and sudden death.

As a pediatrician, I have consistently advocated for vaccines. Although this COVID-19 vaccine is still relatively new, taking it is a no-brainer decision for me. I am aware that there may be side effects, but as a frontline healthcare worker who sees patients nearly daily and is over the age of sixty-five, I believe the benefits of taking this vaccine far outweigh the risks. The correct decision for me is to take it, but every person must make this decision for themselves. For myself, I will continue to take precautions like handwashing and mask-wearing that were mandated indoors, but I look forward to living my life without fear and knowing that I have some protection from the COVID-19 vaccine.

In other news, my husband, Martin, has been checking out the night skies every evening soon after dusk. We're both anxiously anticipating the evening of December 21, when the two largest planets, Jupiter and Saturn, will both align on top of each other, thus resulting in the rare occurrence of the "Star of Bethlehem." This will be an exciting moment to witness, as this night sky event has not been seen in almost eight centuries.

Finally, as I look back on 2020, I realize that my survival through the pandemic was only possible because of my faith. God continues to sustain me and give me strength and hope for better times to come. As one of His children, I will continue to pray and trust that He hears me and already knows what I need even before I ask.

> *"Come and see what the Lord has done, the desolations he has brought on the earth. He makes wars cease to the ends of the earth. He breaks the bow and shatters the spear; he burns the shields with fire. He says, 'Be still, and know that I am God. I will be exalted among the nations; I will be exalted in the earth.' The Lord Almighty is with us; the God of Jacob is our fortress."*
>
> —PSALMS 46:8–11

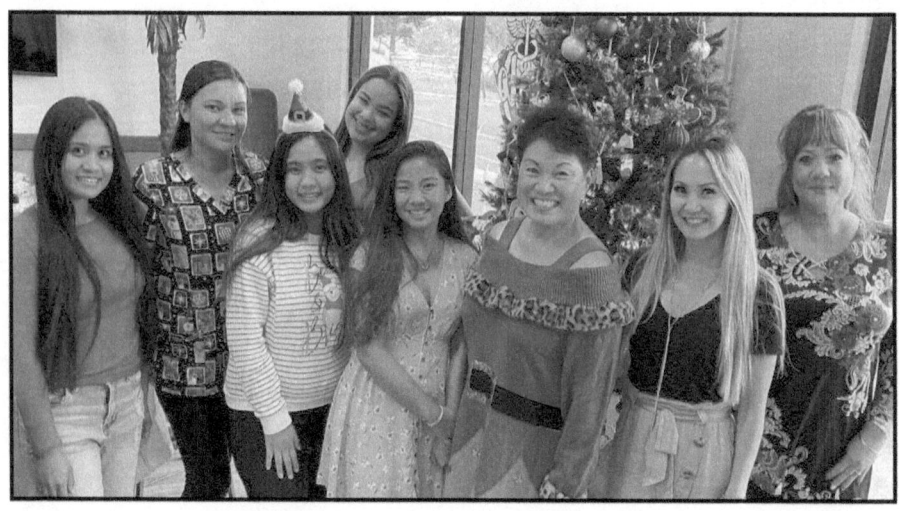

Happy Monday, dear readers!

Just four more days till Christmas. Today, I wanted to have a serious discussion about what is going on right now.

Our front-page headlines revealed a recent rise in the number of active COVID-19 infections, and thus, the possibility of us reverting to Tier 1, according to our mayor. As he said in his own words, opening and shutting down again is hugely dangerous. Despite this, our leaders continue to welcome more tourists each day to Hawaii, but is this the wisest decision at this time? If we shut down again, this will be the third time we have done so, and we may never fully recover for years to come.

In the meantime, the COVID-19 vaccine has arrived in Oahu, and as a frontline healthcare worker, I'm scheduled to receive my vaccine in two days. However, for the public, it will still be a while, if they even consent to getting the COVID-19 vaccine. Current polls show that over 50 percent of the general population have already decided they're not going to take it or are extremely hesitant about it.

New and active COVID-19 numbers are still high, our economy is worsening, but most importantly, the physical and mental health of everyone is continuing to spiral downward. I hear stories daily from the families I see in my office about the many hardships and consequences this virus has brought to everyone. Every day, the solution clearly appears to be worse than the disease itself, and we keep following the marching orders given to us, like sheep going to slaughter.

I understand that this is a new virus and a pandemic that took all of us by surprise, but some of the mandated rules imposed on us seem nonsensical. I was recently in some of the "big box stores" and malls, and they were packed with Christmas shoppers. Most folks were not socially distancing, and the self-checkout machines were not being sanitized after use. We also went out to dine a few times, and our home addresses were no longer required before sitting down. I feel like folks are getting "COVID-19 fatigued" and letting things slide through. I anticipate our numbers will soon be hitting the roof.

Yet, the orders this Christmas are to cancel any gatherings of more than five people and to obey our elected officials. As an American, I'm feeling very frustrated as I see my freedoms slowly slipping away. Even my free speech was recently censored by Facebook, "Big Tech" social media, when I expressed displeasure with rules put out by officials.

Recently, a national panel of expert physicians collectively spoke out in favor of a simple COVID-19 treatment, which included early intervention with the inexpensive combination of Hydroxychloroquine and Zinc. These doctors were silenced, ostracized, and, in some cases, even fired for speaking up on effective early treatment for this virus. Big Pharma, politicians, and other leaders did not want to hear about this, so they immediately condemned it.

So, my question to all of you is, how will you react to what is happening around you? It seems that common sense has gone out the window, and I believe we can no longer remain silent. Please be careful with the general media information being fed to you and keep searching for the "truth." Get educated, ask questions, consider the source of your information, and stay informed about what's happening in our country. I'm feeling a swell of emotions, and I want to reclaim my rights and freedom and return to America I once knew.

I know I'm only one voice in the masses, but if you join me, the silent majority, we can once again rise and make it right.

Tonight is the night to get out and look up at the night sky to check out the "Star of Bethlehem." This was the light that led the Three Wise Men to Bethlehem, where our Lord Jesus Christ was born in a manger more than 2,000 years ago.

Join me tonight in seeking this beautiful light, as the Magi did, to find Him.

> *"After Jesus was born in Bethlehem in Judea, during the time of King Herod, Magi from the East came to Jerusalem and asked, 'Where is the one who has been born king of the Jews? We saw his star when it rose and have come to worship him.'"*

—MATTHEW 2:1–2 NIV

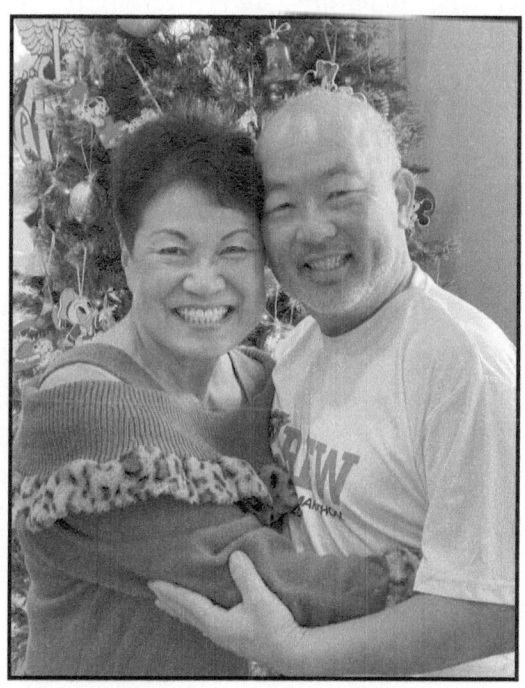

Tonight is Christmas Eve, and Christians worldwide celebrate the greatest gift God gave us: The life, death, and resurrection of our Lord Jesus Christ.

2020 is ending, and it couldn't come soon enough. The COVID-19 virus is getting its "second wind" worldwide and even mutating in some countries. As a frontline healthcare worker, I received my COVID-19 vaccine yesterday and feel very fortunate to have had this priority. So far, so good after twenty-four hours… just a persistent soreness at the injection site on my arm, which Tylenol has helped.

Today, I wanted to share a message of hope as we look forward to 2021, which is just a few days away. God never said life would be easy for any of us, Christians included. During this pandemic, we're all feeling uncertainty, which quickly leads us to fear. However, God reminds us in the Bible that He is in control, even when everything around us seems to be spinning out of control. He is our peace and comfort, and

He knows what He is doing. His ways and everything He allows are so much higher and better than ours. He is aware of all that is happening, all that has happened, and all that will happen. We do not need to fear when we have God in charge of our tomorrows.

When Mary and Joseph were first summoned to be the parents of Jesus, they were initially confused and hesitant but eventually accepted the task after each received an angelic visit. They had no idea what this task they were taking on would entail, but they trusted and persevered, despite many hardships and suffering. They indeed fixed their eyes on God and took that step of faith, without ever looking back.

In the same way, we all need to do the same thing…. On This Christmas Eve, let us reflect on all the blessings God has bestowed upon each of us. There is so much hope in God and with His birth, for by coming to Earth, our sins have been forgiven and washed away. During this Holiday season, remember that no matter what you are going through, God is always with you.

While this holiday season is going to look very different from previous years due to the COVID-19 pandemic, we can all still focus on the reason for the season – the birth of our Lord and Savior, Jesus Christ.

"Suddenly a great company of the heavenly host appeared with the angel, praising God and saying, 'Glory to god in the highest heaven, and on earth peace to those on whom favor rests.' When the angels had left them and gone into heaven, the shepherds said to one another, 'Let's go to Bethlehem and see this thing that has happened which the Lord has told us about."

—LUKE 2:13–15 NIV

Have a Merry Christmas, dear readers.

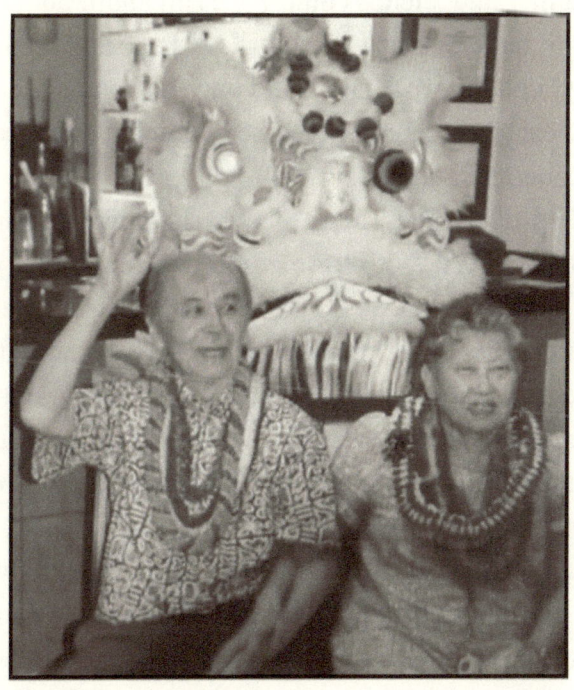

Greetings, dear readers!

Yesterday was a somber day for me. My dear Uncle Robert died after just a brief six-day period with the COVID-19 infection. My Uncle was ninety-three years old and living at a nursing home on Oahu. He was found to have a positive COVID-19 test on 12/23/20 but thankfully exhibited no symptoms. The administration decided to transfer him for observation to Wahiawa General Hospital the next morning. For the ensuing six days, I received a daily email from my cousin, who reported that he was doing excellently, with no fever or other symptoms and even continued to have an excellent appetite.

Then, suddenly, to my utter surprise, yesterday's email noted that he had taken a sudden turn for the worse, and his oxygen level was dropping drastically. It went on to say that it was clear he would not survive the day. He was not allowed to have any visitors with him, and he passed away in the afternoon alone.

I felt so sad and upset at this. The hospital placed an iPad on his bed so that family and friends could FaceTime him, but of course, this was just not the same as being with our loved one and holding his hand. Unfortunately, I had to work and could only hop on FaceTime intermittently. By the early afternoon, I received an email announcing that my dear Uncle Robert had passed.

My Uncle Robert and Aunty Nora, along with their three children, have always been there for me and my family. They lived three houses away from me, and we all grew up together. I remember having Wednesday night dinners every week with them, along with my maternal grandparents and the entire family. My mom and grandfather would spend the whole day making the most unusual and delectable Chinese dishes. It was always so much fun to get together at midweek for a big family meal.

Additionally, Uncle Robert and Aunty Nora would always include us in special events, such as the movie musicals at the then-brand-new Cinerama Theater, with its surround sound and state-of-the-art screens. What a treat this was for us.

One of my fondest memories of childhood was their annual Christmas Day dinner party, which Uncle Robert and Aunty Nora put on year after year. I recall attending this event from the time I was a little girl, and it became my favorite, most anticipated annual Christmas tradition. When I was a little girl, the party was at their home, but as the family grew larger, they began to have parties at restaurants. Relatives from the mainland would even fly in to attend this special event. I always found this celebration was the perfect time to catch up with relatives that I had not seen or rarely spoken to throughout the year. We always played Bingo, the "Price Is Right" game, as well as guessing contests with prizes galore. We ended the gala by gathering in a large circle, and each person had a wrapped Christmas gift to exchange. The music would start, and when it ended, that was your grab bag gift. We always ended the evening singing "Hawaii Aloha" – so many great memories!

2020 was the first year that the annual Christmas Day dinner party had to be cancelled, but the many memories made will be cherished forever.

Today, let's pause and reflect on how precious our time is in this world. No one knows how much time God will allow us here, but let's all live life as if it were our last day. Take the time during this Holiday Season to reach out to family, friends, and even strangers and make a positive difference in their lives today. Your small gesture will send out ripples of kindness, and your legacy of love will live on in the lives you have touched.

Thank you, Uncle Robert, for the gentle and loving ways you always supported me.

> *"For God so loved the world that he gave his one and only Son, that whoever believes in him shall not perish but have eternal life."*
>
> —JOHN 3:16 NIV

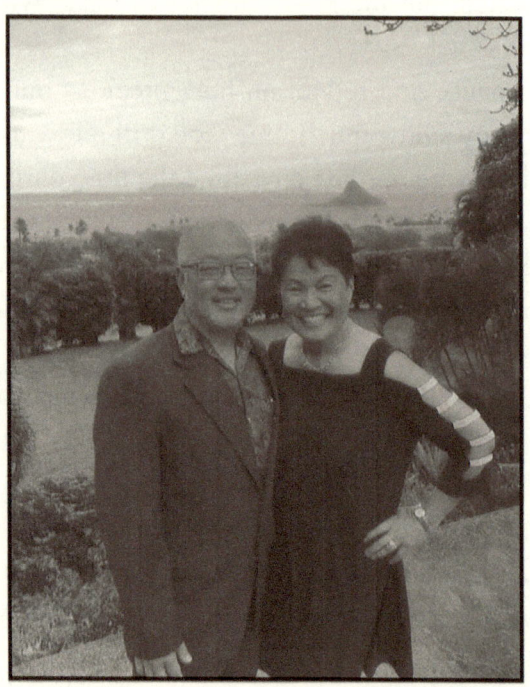

H appy New Year's Eve! Today will be the final entry for 2020. This past year has been a year for history books. It has been quite a rollercoaster ride for me. Everyone has been affected in some way by the COVID-19 pandemic. For 2021, I feel we all need to be kinder and more compassionate to ourselves as we consider our goals for the coming year.

Traditionally, currently, many of us have started making huge goals for ourselves or our businesses. Whatever goals you're considering, think about smaller, bite-sized ones and allow yourself to make a few mistakes. In looking back on this year, one thing has become quite evident to me: Plans and circumstances can and will change frequently and without notice. As a result, the silver lining to all the uncertainties was learning to be flexible and adapt to the many challenges constantly being thrown my way.

I recently ran across an excellent article by Omar Itani entitled *Why You Need to Embrace This 'One Day at a Time' Philosophy* which I thought was very appropriate to share with you today. This concept is simple and helps direct our attention to what we can do today because that's the only place in time we can control. This concept is essential to remember because in times like these, we all need to feel a bit in control of our lives and learn to focus on the current moments in front of us.

It is futile to spend our precious time and energy dwelling on the past because yesterday is gone. We need to reflect and learn from the past, then move on. The future, on the other hand, has not yet arrived. We can obsess about future dreams and goals, but if we don't act today, we'll never be able to reach them.

Therefore, for 2021, the most critical question we should be asking ourselves daily is, "What can I do today that will move me one step closer to my goals?" We each have the power to make choices that can transform our lives, but we can only do it one day at a time.

No one knows what 2021 will bring, but let's keep reminding ourselves to live one day at a time. I recently came across a quote that reads, "Success is the product of daily habits."

So, dear readers, family, and friends, keep your chin up, continue to persevere, and never give up. Take those small steps consistently over time, and eventually, you will find yourself creating a significant difference in your future.

As we start the New Year, one of my goals will be to read the Bible and turn to God in prayer daily. We can always find hope and encouragement in God's word, so I hope you will consider doing the same.

Happy New Year to all of you and may God continue to bless each of you abundantly along your life's journey.

> *"Rejoice in the Lord always. I will repeat it: Rejoice! Let your gentleness be evident to all. The Lord is nearby. Do not be anxious about anything, but in every situation by prayer and petition, with thanksgiving, present your requests to God."*

—PHILIPPIANS 4:4–6 NIV

ABOUT THE AUTHOR

Dr. Theresa Wee is a practicing pediatrician, wellness expert, and a mother of four. She has devoted her life to helping others by sharing her expertise as a healthcare professional, but also by sharing her trials as a human being. She has a strong commitment to improving the health of the people of Hawaii and began her non-profit organization, "Walk with a Doc – Oahu," in 2016. She lives with her husband Martin in Hawaii. In her spare time, she enjoys traveling and spending time with her five grandchildren. Her hobbies include water aerobics, hiking, and cooking.

www.ingramcontent.com/pod-product-compliance
Lightning Source LLC
Chambersburg PA
CBHW020414150626
46554CB00014B/1235